THE
HAPPY,
HEALTHY
REVOLUTION

THE WORKING PARENT'S GUIDE TO ACHIEVE WELLNESS AS A FAMILY

THERESA Y. WEE, M.D.

Ordering Information:

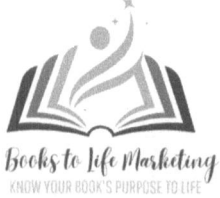

Books to Life Marketing Ltd
128 City Road, London, EC1V 2NX, UK

Printed in the United States of America

CONTENTS

Advance Praise v
Foreword xi

Chapter 1: Family Health in Jeopardy. 1
Chapter 2: Working Parents Need Help Now –
            I Get It. 10
Chapter 3: Thinking Outside the Box in
            Today's World 25
Chapter 4: Family Teamwork Is the Key to
            Success 32
Chapter 5: Nourishing Our Bodies Daily 42
Chapter 6: Move More 60
Chapter 7: The Incredible Value of Sleep and
            Family Meals 72
Chapter 8: Small Goals Amount to Big Wins .. 80
Chapter 9: Life Is About Being in the Present
            Moment 88
Chapter 10: A Positive Attitude Changes
            Everything. 94
Chapter 11: Keep the Passion Burning 100
Chapter 12: Oops, We Are Only Human 107
Chapter 13: Exceptional Family Health for Life. . 115

Acknowledgments 121
About the Author 125
Thank You 127

ADVANCE PRAISE

"As a friend and colleague for twenty years, I know that Theresa practices what she preaches. *The Happy, Healthy Revolution* doesn't just identify America's problems of obesity and family dysfunction, but more importantly demonstrates practical ways to solve them. If you put into practice what she preaches, it will lead to a healthy, well balanced lifestyle that will bring joy to you and your family each day."

—*John H. Houk, MD, FACP*, John A. Burns School of Medicine Assistant Clinical Professor

"Theresa's holistic approach to wellness is both refreshing and effective. It is grounded in personal experience and perfectly reflects Hawaii values. This book should be considered a roadmap to good health for families nationwide."

—*Josh Green MD*, Hawaii Lieutenant Governor

"It is an honor to have supported Theresa Y. Wee MD through AlohaCare's Waiwai Ola Community grant in the recent year! As a Hawaii pediatrician, she has been caring for our keiki and families, and her expertise has impacted her approach to preventing and treating obesity in Hawaii through an innovative family approach. *The Happy Healthy Revolution* is based on Dr. Wee's Family Workshops from the Waiwai Ola Grant. Her plan for healthy living helps people to see that each day counts."

—*Carol Sato*, AlohaCare Care Strategy Director

"Dr. Theresa Wee walks beside us, sharing her life's journey and weaving insightful expertise and sage guidance in *The Happy, Healthy Revolution*. If you ever felt alone or discouraged as a parent—hang on—hope is here.

—*Danny Yamashiro*, Radio Host of The Good Life Hawaii 99.5 KGU-FM

"Growing up in Hawaii, Dr. Wee embraced 'working hard' as one of her core values from her family of origin. In *The Happy, Healthy Revolution*, she exposes how the same will can sometimes threaten family values. From her own experience, Dr. Wee offers insights on how to balance 'doing' and 'being' in order to achieve a sense of well-being. The most practical and most valuable piece of work for our much-needed present context."

—*Rev.JP Sabbithi, D.Min Pastor*, Joy of Christ Lutheran Church, Pearl City, Hawaii.

For Stephen L. Wee. MD

You are so loved and missed, but your legacy of compassion and service to others lives on. Thank you for being such a wonderful husband, father, and physician. You have positively touched and changed the lives of many in your brief lifetime.

FOREWORD

When Dr. Wee shared she was writing a book, I told our Walk with a Doc team, "This is fantastic. This is exactly who should be sharing how it is done!" Then, she asked if I would be willing to write the foreword. It is an honor. After reading the final product, I was, once again, so proud of Theresa. She has nailed something that is so critically important to us all.

Dr. Wee gets "it." As individuals, we all have the power to prevent, treat, or cure so many of the problems that can interrupt our daily lives. Yet, often we need someone to guide us through that tunnel. Dr. Wee does that for us.

Theresa's passion for others is on grand display as she leads us through the ins and outs of getting those simple, small wins that all add up to change our lives in a big, big way. I am so grateful that Dr. Wee took the time to share with us all what has made her a raging success with her patients, their families, and her community.

Nothing is more important than our health. Theresa, thank you from the bottom of my heart for being such a beacon of light and getting it all down in this wonderful book. You are a gift to us all!

With great respect,

David Sabgir, M.D.
Cardiologist C.E.O. and
Founder—Walk with a Doc

CHAPTER 1

FAMILY HEALTH IN JEOPARDY

As a young girl growing up in Hawaii in the sixties, I believed in fairy tales, happy endings, and dreams always coming true. My parents told me I could be anything I wanted, and the world was bursting with great opportunities, even for women. Although my mom was a licensed social worker with a master's degree, she became a stay-at-home mom after having all four of us children. I was determined to complete everything.

I discovered my calling at seven after reading the autobiography of the first woman to become a doctor, Elizabeth Blackwell. Only a few women physicians were in Hawaii in the sixties, but her story inspired me. In addition to wanting to be a doctor, I wanted to be married and have a family, preferably with four children.

The Struggles of Working Mothers

As the years unfolded, and with much hard work, effort, and perseverance, I achieved these goals, including having four children. As a full-time, practicing pediatrician and working mom, I quickly discovered that I, too, was struggling to juggle the constant demands and details that come with working both in and outside the home. Although "women's liberation" and equal rights were significant topics, childcare and household matters were still considered women's primary responsibilities.

Early in my pediatric practice, I encountered working mothers who were stretched to the limit, chronically tired, and doing their best to balance their responsibilities both at home and work. They had no time to buy groceries or prepare a healthy meal every night. Instead, they defaulted on fast food or takeout pizza and wrestled with a guilty conscience for the rest of the evening.

The weekends are the time for these mothers to catch up on all the household chores, but unfortunately, this leaves no time for themselves, their husbands, or their families. In the meantime, Dad is also busy with his "Dad duties," like yard work, house repairs, "honey-do lists," or working his second, part-time job. As a result, husbands and wives have no time to connect or their children. They both feel stressed and believe they are doing their best to survive the week.

Every day in the office, I see this lack of time for recharging, resulting in many marriages eroding, children with behavioral and mental health problems, confusion, and chaos within the family unit. Initially, as a young pediatrician, I was shocked to see how minor disagreements gradually evolved into monumental challenges and conflict within families over time.

During my medical school and residency training, I received thorough instruction on physical illnesses, diseases, treatments, and medications. Still, I was not prepared to address the many challenges families, parents, and children were starting to face in this new era of technology, fast food, mental illness, and social isolation.

As the years went on and newer, more effective vaccines became available, I no longer saw as many critically ill children as I had during my pediatric residency training in the early 1980s. Admitting children to our pediatric hospital was soon becoming a rare event, but now, a new epidemic is starting to take place. I am now seeing the slow dissolution of the family unit. Family conflicts, dysfunction, and breakups are becoming increasingly common.

New Emerging Trend of Obesity in All Ages

One of the first concerning trends I noticed was the rapid rise of more children becoming overweight or obese. They were slowly developing unhealthy habits, primarily due to their parents not having the time, energy, or resources for preparing healthier home-cooked meals. Costco and fast-food establishments became the choice for my parents, who were also gaining weight and developing unhealthy habits. Family meals became scarce, and communication among the family diminished significantly. Additionally, the era of technology and increased screen time appears to promote social isolation and distance among individuals, as well as between them and their surroundings. Children are becoming increasingly less physically active and often spend most of their time indoors, using their phones, playing video games, or watching Netflix or TV. My patients' mothers would usually express to me their deep frustration that they failed because they could not provide as much home-cooked food, family activities, and quality time with their children as they wanted. As these mothers confided in me about their frustration, I quietly acknowledged that I understood every word they said because that was exactly what I was experiencing and feeling. I, too, was a full-time working mother and felt the heavy burden of both roles.

Many parents, both mothers and fathers, would tell me that their schedules were filled with numerous mundane tasks to complete each day. They yearned for simpler times when the family did more spontaneous activities together, like when they were growing up. I slowly began to see more parents going on crash diets or getting gym memberships at expensive health clubs to get back on track, but these plans inevitably failed. Today's parents are pulled in all directions and often neglect their health.

Social media nowadays offers answers to any of our questions at the click of a button. Some may be true, but much of the information is also misleading. My parents and my teenage patients often ask me about the latest trends in popular diets or workouts to help them improve their health. I tell everyone that none of these quick fixes will ever work, and if they did, I would hear about these amazing breakthroughs in my medical journals. In today's world of instant gratification, we seem increasingly willing to spend our money on quick fixes, but we often end up back where we started, regaining all or even some of the weight.

As my practice grew over the years, I became acutely aware of how prevalent this feeling of families losing control, gaining more weight, and becoming unhealthier was. It was an unspoken, quiet desperation of hopelessness, and it felt like everyone in the family was destined for deteriorating health and family disconnectedness.

My Struggles

As a full-time working mother of four young children, I faced the same challenges and frustrations in my own family. After being in private practice for a few years, taking time off or going on vacation from my six-day workweek became difficult. We had a mortgage, private school tuition, preschool, daycare, and sustaining all the costs of running our new private practices. In fact, after having my last two children, I returned to work within days after giving birth. Life was not easy then; sometimes, you do what you must.

I truly knew what my working moms were feeling, and my heart ached for all the families struggling with this dilemma of two working parents trying their best to get things in order. Earlier generations of parents never had to face these issues because most mothers stayed at home. I wanted families to be harmonious and happy again, even with two working parents. They, too, deserved that daily family time and connectedness. I wanted to show others that this could be done somehow. Thus, this marked the beginning of my new journey to find ways to unite my family and other families, making them stronger, happier, and healthier.

I honestly believe that the answer to carrying out this goal is to get everyone in the family to understand why it is so urgent to work together, as well as the many rewards they will reap once they embark on this life-changing process. After conducting workshop sessions for families with obese and overweight children for many years, I could see that not only would parents enjoy a multitude of benefits from leading healthier lifestyles, but the children and the grandparents would also experience positive changes if they were all in with the program from the start.

The Importance of the Family Unit

The idea of involving the entire family is the secret ingredient of this revolutionary program, and I'm excited to share the solution I stumbled upon. It worked in our home, and I knew it could help the families I saw daily in similar situations. Of course, making lasting changes would require commitment, time, patience, and persistence from all family members. This is not a quick-fix plan, but I guarantee it will help restore fun, laughter, better health, and unity for you and your family. Now, do you not want to be a part of this program?

As a pediatrician, I began to realize the importance of the family unit in the overall well-being of both parents and children. The family is the most important influence in a child's life, and those childhood years are crucial for their development. Children need to feel the love and security of the family and have a sense of belonging.

I am always amazed that anyone can become a parent without training or preparation. We, as parents, strive to do our best, but we are just imitating what we remember our parents doing. However, most mothers of the earlier generation did not face the stress of working a full-time job outside the home.

Somehow, it seems imperative that a new model or shift in thinking of shared responsibility in the home evolves. Now, more than ever, the traditional roles of moms and dads must be redefined. Moreover, this may not be enough in today's busy world. Another key ingredient of healthy living and family harmony is engaging children, preferably from an early age, to contribute to the daily life of the family.

As I continued to work within my own family and other families in my practice, I could see that things could improve with just a few simple changes and a bit of patience. This simple program is a proven way to reap enormous benefits of better health for the entire household through minor modifications, and it is tailored to overcome your hectic schedules. The family unit can be strengthened again, and everyone will be eager to return to their home oasis in the evening. That is my hope for you, dear reader, and the reason I am writing this book. I promise you that help is within your reach.

I hope my experience and ability as a pediatrician and mother can help you start on a simple, proven plan to improve your physical and emotional health, as well as that of your husband, children, and parents. As the many benefits unfold, you will see a light at the end of the tunnel, and it is never too late to start.

The tips, tricks, and secrets I have woven throughout this book have proven effective and can change your life and your family's life now.

So, if you're ready, fasten your seatbelts, and let's start this journey today.

CHAPTER 2

WORKING PARENTS NEED HELP NOW – I GET IT

While growing up in the 1960s and 1970s, I began to see a slow, gradual acceptance of women entering medicine, engineering, business, and other traditionally male-dominated occupations. However, many still did not believe that women belonged in these fields. I distinctly recall attending to my assigned premedical advisor as a first-year student at the University of Hawaii, Manoa. The first words out of her mouth were, "I don't think you should go into medicine, and you need to consider another field of interest." I at once grabbed my papers and never went back to her again.

I got my Bachelor of Science in Biology with the highest honors in three years. Additionally, at the tender age of twenty, I gained early acceptance into the University of Hawaii John A. Burns School of

Medicine at the start of my third year in college. I sometimes wonder what would have happened if I had followed that premedical advisor's advice, but I had my family's support, which mattered to me then. Having one or two people in your corner believing in you can make the most significant difference.

My four years as a medical student were challenging and required many hours of study, but we bonded as a class and worked together to support one another through the difficult times. By the process of elimination, I decided that pediatrics would be my specialty.

Meeting and Marrying My "Best" Friend

During my first year as an undergraduate at the University of Hawaii, I was fortunate to make a new friend, Stephen Wee, a pre-medical student. We both hit it off, and he and I were in that "friend zone" for the next seven years. Most of all, he lived close by and always gave me rides in his cute light-blue Volkswagen Beetle. You could say it was a relationship of convenience. He was such a great guy, and I never understood why he never had a girlfriend.

Finally, after seven years of brotherly friendship and free car rides, in our fourth and final year of medical school, he looked at me one evening we were out and said, "I think we should go for it." I replied, "Go for what? Ice cream?" After a few minutes of awkward silence, I finally realized that this was his marriage proposal, and he asked me to marry him. I was caught off guard, but as corny as this sounds, I realized what a genuinely wonderful man he was and knew I had to be with him for the rest of my life. And anyway, I still needed rides and all the thoughtful things he always did for me, without a single complaint. I thought, "Wow, I just won the lottery!"

So, I accepted this unique marriage proposal, and then we started to date. We were married on May 24, 1980, in Honolulu, Hawaii, and off we went to Columbus, Ohio, for our respective residencies. I spent three years as a pediatric intern and resident at Columbus Children's Hospital, now known as Nationwide Children's Hospital, and then did an ambulatory fellowship there. This was followed by two years of finally having my first real job in private practice in Westerville, Ohio, where I gained even more experience as a young primary care pediatrician. Stephen completed his three-year internal medicine residency at Riverside Methodist Hospital and then worked for three years at the emergency room in Lancaster, Ohio.

The Scary Reality of Having Your Child

We had our first child – what a revelation for both of us. My husband, an internal medicine specialist, and I, a trained pediatrician, brought this little bundle of joy home. That first night home, I remember calling my mom in Hawaii and just crying over the phone, saying that I was a scared, inexperienced first-time parent and asking her to catch the next plane over to Ohio to help me. As I look back, this seems silly, mainly as a trained pediatrician, but at the time, the feeling of responsibility and dependence of this baby on me was just so overwhelming. I tell many of the families I work with that I know exactly that feeling of fear and shock at night with their newborn baby. As I have said, my experience of raising four children has been just as valuable as my pediatric residency training.

Four Children, Full-Time Doc, and the Slow Burnout

In 1984, with our second son on the way, we decided it was time to return to Hawaii. There was a new housing development coming up in Central Oahu. Even though this was away from the city and considered "country," we decided to buy a home there because there was a new vacant medical office building just a few blocks up the road. We were the first tenants to lease space there, and in 1984, we installed our signs, officially beginning our combined pediatric and internal medicine practices. It took four years to build our private practices, so for those first few years, we both worked at other part-time jobs as physicians to keep the lights on and pay for daycare, preschool, home mortgages, and everything else.

We had an idyllic life: four healthy, active children, two growing medical practices, flexible hours, and a lovely home. But underneath this façade, I slowly suffocated. I worked six days a week, seeing patients in the office and then taking my work home to finish charting and making phone calls. I was on call twenty-four hours a day, 365 days a year, to handle emergencies. I often commuted to the city to see, admit, and care for my critically ill patients at the Kapiolani Children's Hospital. This job as a pediatrician, caring for other people's children, left me with no energy for my children and my husband at the end of the day. I did not know it at the time, but I was slowly burning out. I told myself *I was a professional woman* and *made it this far. I can excel as both a full-time pediatrician and a dedicated mom at home.*

The Breaking Point at Age Forty

At the age of forty, with four highly active children, all under the age of twelve, I began to experience a gradual decline in my appetite, difficulty falling and staying asleep, a loss of joy in almost everything, and a feeling of a heavy burden on my shoulders, daily. I felt this way for over a year and just barely made it from day to day. My husband and I, both physicians, could not figure out what was wrong with me. I cried often, felt hopeless, and yearned for the day when I could feel myself again.

The daily tasks of a working mom, who also had to keep up with all the responsibilities of a mother of four children, continued despite my feelings, and I had to maintain a happy face. One day, while reading a medical journal, I came across an article on the significant signs of depression, and I finally self-diagnosed myself as depressed. Within a week, I sought the care of an excellent psychiatrist who at once diagnosed me with depression and placed me on two weeks of leave from the office, antidepressants, and weekly therapy. Within weeks, I slowly crawled out of that dark hole and felt like I was once again. I was relieved to see hope finally.

At this point in my life, this episode of depression was a life-changing wake-up call for me. I realized I was not a superwoman and could not do everything alone. I needed to put my pride aside and humbly accept the help and support of my husband, children, parents, and in-laws. We sat down with everyone, including the children, and explained to them what was happening with Their Mom. We discussed the importance of everyone contributing to the family and making contributions based on their age and abilities. My husband also pitched in and helped even more with household chores. My parents and mother-in-law also helped with home-cooked meals, cleaning, occasional childcare, grocery shopping, and more.

Sometimes, the darkest parts of our lives can be the best places to learn. I gained a great deal of insight into how overwhelmed a person can become, and that we must accept help graciously and humbly during certain life seasons. It was also a challenging learning experience, but I believe this has made me a better mother and a more compassionate doctor. I could relate to my working parents and the trials they faced daily. I would not want to go through this again, but the lessons I learned from this challenging situation have stayed with me for life and enriched my life even more.

The Banner Year of 2010

2010 was a banner year for me. My husband and I celebrated our thirtieth wedding anniversary with a two-week trip to China. This was our first time taking an overseas trip, and it was a truly memorable and well-deserved vacation. We reminisced on the last thirty years of demanding work and looked forward to the next thirty years of married bliss and time together as empty nesters. The three older boys had graduated from college, and the youngest, our daughter, had just turned twenty-one years old and was moving on to her final year at Westmont College in Santa Barbara. However, God had other plans in store for us.

On Friday, June 11, 2010, my husband, best friend, and business partner died suddenly and unexpectedly in my arms within minutes. We had just returned from our memorable vacation two weeks earlier, and after seeing our morning patients, my husband told me he was not feeling well. I did not think anything about this comment and told him that I would heat our lunches and be back. A few minutes later, when I returned with our lunch, he was dead.

He was only fifty-five years old and had no known medical problems until then. He had just seen his primary care physician and had a clean bill of health. According to the autopsy report, he had an aortic aneurysm that ruptured. For the first few weeks, I went into utter shock and disbelief. I was numb, mad, sad, confused, and experiencing all kinds of emotions at once. In addition to all of this, the real estate management company informed me that my office lease was up in two weeks and that they were going to more than double my rent, requiring me to sign a lease for a term of at least five or ten years. I declined to sign these terms, so they gave me one year to vacate.

My Answer from God

At this point in my life, I could have quit medicine and retired completely, which my four grown children vigorously encouraged me to do. However, there was something inside of me that kept saying it was not my time to quit medicine at the age of fifty-four years. I continued seeing my patients in the office, and several of my husband's colleagues continued to help and see his patients as well, graciously. My practice was slowly going bankrupt, and I knew I had to vacate my office in a year. Things did not look good at all; in fact, they looked hopeless. My world had turned upside down, and it felt as if someone had ripped half of my heart out. My husband was the one and only real boyfriend I had, and now I was alone. Who am I? What is my purpose in life now? I had a lot to sort out. In the meantime, I had stopped attending church and felt so much anger toward God for taking my husband and business partner at such an early age.

One night, three months after my husband's sudden death, I went down on my knees and desperately cried out to God: "Please show me a sign about what you want me to do!" I waited for an answer, and within five days, I received a call from someone referred to me by another physician, who stated that she had twenty years of experience as an office practice manager. She asked me to meet with her and offered to help with my business. Could this be the sign from God I so desperately needed?

When she arrived, she told me I looked so distraught that she felt compelled to offer her services for free until I could get back on my feet again, to pay her back. She looked me in the eyes and told me she could turn my practice around, but before we went any further, she requested permission to pray for me. The only thought that came to mind when she said this was that it was indeed the sign from God that I had requested a few days ago.

She started work immediately in my office and made the necessary changes to help my new practice achieve a turnaround. We renamed my practice "Wee Pediatrics, Inc." and began vigorously rebuilding it. I was fortunate to find a brand-new, empty office space for sale nearby, which is double the size of my previous office. I decided to buy it, and only through the grace of God did the loans go through. I began designing, planning, and constructing my new office.

In December 2011, just eighteen months after my husband's death, I moved into my newly constructed office, the Wee Wellness Center. This was the start of a new chapter as a business owner and solo practitioner, and I knew God had more plans in store for me.

Fulfilling My Passion in Life

About a month after I started working for myself, my office manager turned to me and asked a question that no one had ever asked me before: "What is your passion?" I replied immediately that my passion had always been to help working mothers and their families stay healthy, prevent obesity, and strengthen the all-important family unit. This, coincidentally, was also a deep personal passion for her. She had three daughters, and as a single mother for most of her life, she needed to work two to three jobs to support them. She had concerns, like other working mothers, about providing the best meals and parenting her children to the best of her ability with her limited time. Thus, in 2011, my office manager and I began free in-office workshops for my families with obese and overweight children who were ready for change. The families that took part had to agree to have the entire family attend five two-hour Saturday afternoon sessions. My office manager, staff, other volunteers, an army recruiter, and I conducted these in my lobby. We did several cohorts over the next few years, yielding incredibly positive results. As my practice got busier, these workshops eventually had to be postponed due to time constraints. However, I knew that many families still needed help.

Walk with a Doc – Oahu

In February 2016, with the help of UHA Health Insurance and its CEO, Howard Lee, I launched a chapter of the nonprofit organization Walk with a Doc – Oahu, which allowed me to reach out to my entire community for a free weekly walking event. I invited people of all ages, fitness levels, and insurance backgrounds to join me for a walk in Central Oahu Regional Park, near the tennis courts, on Saturday from 8:00 to 9:00 a.m. for health, fellowship, and fun. This free weekly event began in 2016, but soon word began to spread in the community, and we now have thirty to forty walkers each week. I share a new health tip weekly, and then we stretch, walk for forty-five minutes, and finally cool down, followed by water and fruit refreshments generously donated by Stay Fit Physical Therapy.

Earlier this year, we were able to kick off a new chapter of Walk with a Future Doc at the Kakaako Waterfront Park every fourth Sunday. This is organized by our enthusiastic University of Hawaii John A. Burns School of Medicine (JABSOM) medical students and faculty, who also recognize the value that community involvement can bring to everyone. We have recently established additional programs, including Hike with a Doc, Dance with a Doc, Craft with a Doc, and Cook with a Doc. These programs aim to reinforce the social connections formed, teach a new skill, and help everyone become more active together in different venues. Social interactions and knowing you are not alone on this journey towards better health make all the difference. Over the past years, I have heard many excellent testimonials and seen positive physical and emotional results from my walkers. Every week, someone would come up to me with tears in their eyes to tell me that this was just that little nudge they needed to embark on their journey toward better health. As my walkers become healthier, I have seen some move on to other activities, such as playing pickleball, traveling the world, or participating in half-marathons. As a physician leader for Walk with a Doc- Oahu, I feel delighted knowing I made a small contribution to improving someone's health. I also thank my walkers for keeping me accountable for my health. There are many Saturdays when I don't feel like getting up and going, but I know my walkers expect me. After taking the walk, I feel exhilarated and ready for the weekend. As my son recently reminded me, "Hey, Mom, you cannot become obese because you are the Walk with a Doc leader."

In early 2019, I was fortunate enough to receive a grant from the Aloha Care Community Intervention Program Wai Wai Ola Program. As a result of this, I was able to restart my workshop sessions for families with obese or overweight children. I conducted three cohorts, each with five to six families, and named my program the Hawaii Healthy Family Revolution. The results of our intervention for the three family cohorts are in, and they show not only positive physical benefits, such as decreased weight, percent body fat, and waist circumference, but also, most remarkably, positive mental benefits, including improved emotional well-being and improved depression scores in most of our participants. Additionally, 100 percent of the families felt ready and able to use the information obtained in this program to help with planning and decision-making for improving their health and that of their children.

The Hawaii Healthy Family Revolution Gains National Recognition

On September 8, 2019, I was honored to present my Hawaii Healthy Family Revolution Program nationally at the 2019 Patient-Centered Medical Home Congress held in Boston, Massachusetts. It was a great honor to share this with like-minded colleagues across the nation. It was very well received, and I will follow up with national groups, such as the Centers for Disease Control. I was invited to speak at the 2020 International Obesity Chronic Disease Conference (IOCDC) on July 6, 2020, in San Francisco to present my family workshops internationally. However, this in-person conference was canceled due to the COVID-19 pandemic.

We plan to contact companies or groups interested in making this program available to their employees. Additionally, I would like to continue these workshops for families ready for change and extend them to adults and seniors. Soon, I would like to approach health insurance companies and have them help cover the cost of participation in innovative programs like this. Our families desperately need help now, especially our children. This would be an amazing win-win situation, not only for health insurance companies in the future but also for preserving the family unit and promoting the health of people of all ages, thereby maintaining it.

I continue to serve as the Medical Director of Wee Pediatrics, Inc., and am assisted by another pediatrician, Dr. Jordan Arakawa, and a pediatric nurse practitioner, Myrtle Parel, who both help me see patients in the office daily.

For the past five years, I have also had the honor and pleasure of providing a monthly health tip on a local morning news program, "Living 808," on KHON. Additionally, I have appeared in numerous guest segments on radio shows, including HPR's The Body Show and the Kupuna Wiki radio show, and have delivered *in-person* presentations to various community groups.

My goal for the coming years is to continue developing innovative solutions to help and encourage the people of Hawaii to lead healthier lives. My hope and dream are that people will realize that health is their most incredible wealth and that it is never too late to start this journey.

CHAPTER 3

THINKING OUTSIDE THE BOX IN TODAY'S WORLD

As a student in the sixties, my parents enrolled me in a popular speed-reading course called Evelyn Wood's Reading Dynamics. I'm not sure if I learned how to speed read, but one takeaway that has been extremely valuable for the rest of my life is always to preview or scan the book from front to back, look at the table of contents, and understand what I want to get from reading the book.

In this chapter, I aim to provide you with an overview of the program, enabling you to understand this unique approach to better health for you and your entire family. The first and most important basis for success is the buy-in and enthusiastic participation of all family members in the household. It is an all-or-nothing deal. What I have found over the years is that if anyone resists, the family will have much more difficulty succeeding. If most of the family is on board, try giving the naysayer a gentle "nudge" and asking that person to at least try it. Once you start, it's hard to stop, and soon the whole family is having a great time. Another suggestion would be to discuss this with your primary care physician and see if they can give this family member a little "nudge" of encouragement.

The whole idea of this program is to encourage the entire family to develop healthy habits for a lifetime, so we certainly cannot leave a household member behind. I will provide you with basic information about nutrition and exercise in an easy-to-understand manner, along with tools that your entire family can use immediately to achieve your goals.

There is an overwhelming amount of information online about which new diets or exercises are the most effective, which can confuse everyone, including physicians. I will simplify the information I share with you on food and exercise so that you will clearly understand the many choices available.

Making Changes for a Lifetime

For anyone to make lifestyle changes, it is essential to implement them gradually over time so that they become a lifelong habit. A lot valuable information will be presented, but I intend for you and your family to sit down and make a joint decision, one small bit at a time. I will provide you with tools to use as a family, but you must choose the one simple change you and your family would like to start with.

My Plate and 5210

You will learn basic nutritional information, including the valuable MyPlate illustration and the 5-2-1-0 concept, to help you gradually adopt healthier habits. I will also discuss one of the major causes of excessive weight gain in the United States today: the consumption of sugar-sweetened beverages. Nowadays, wherever you go, whether it's a fast-food chain, a restaurant, a party, or simply at home, the menus and refrigerators are filled with these sugar-sweetened beverages. Most places allow you to have unlimited amounts of these beverages or super-size them for the same price as a small one. In my experience teaching families in my workshop, I have found that this topic is the most popular and eye-opening takeaway lesson they learn.

Family Awareness of Sleep and Family Meals

Additionally, many other factors come into play when discussing the control of weight gain, low energy, and chronic fatigue. The two most crucial factors will be discussed in detail: sleep and family meals. These critical factors help individuals maintain a healthy weight and prevent weight gain over time. I will share ideas on diverse ways you and your family can successfully achieve adequate sleep and be available for family meals, which are always challenges for many families.

Since this is a family-based program, I will emphasize the importance of involving children of all ages in planning, preparing, and cooking meals. This gets everyone involved, and the kids can take pride in and ownership of what they have helped prepare. This will lead to more family connections, and everyone will be more likely to eat the healthy meals they helped create.

One of the crucial steps in this program is understanding that screen time is a great robbery of personal and family time. You will know that the sooner you set boundaries and rules as parents on screen time, the more the children are likely to comply. We refer to this as a media plan, a discussion that must be ongoing and adjusted based on the child's age and needs. It is also essential that parents or guardians adhere to these guidelines so that the children can see consistency being maintained.

Setting Goals

The following important chapter equips you with tools for setting and achieving small family goals. For any habit to become part of your routine, you must do it for thirty days. You will learn to use the S.M.A.R.T. approach, and each part of this approach is detailed and taught to you in an easy-to-understand manner.

Once the program is in full swing, everyone in the household must hold each other accountable and work toward shared family goals. Additionally, I will discuss the importance of setting consistent mealtimes, bedtimes, family routines, and schedules, and adhering to them. By keeping everyone "on track," success as a family is inevitable with time and patience.

Be Present in the Moment

Two valuable concepts are introduced in the program: the essential roles of mindfulness and meditation. Today's world is hectic, and everything around us moves at a rapid pace. However, in the rush to complete our work by multitasking, we may lose touch with the present situation. We are missing what we are doing or what we are feeling. Mindfulness is the practice of purposely focusing on the present moment and accepting it without judgment. Numerous recent studies have demonstrated that mindfulness offers multiple health benefits, including reducing stress and promoting happiness. I will teach basic mindfulness meditation, a popular method of focusing on your breathing or other bodily sensations.

Being Grateful Always

Ultimately, we will explore the benefits of gratitude for the well-being and success of everyone. Gratitude is about feeling and expressing appreciation for all that you have received. This is a skill worth developing, as it can significantly change your perspective on life. There is always something to be grateful for, no matter how many negative things keep coming at you. Gratitude helps us stop focusing on day-to-day annoyances and instead lets us see more clearly the abundance in our lives. Study after study shows the benefits of practicing and journaling gratitude, which positively impact our physical and emotional well-being, strengthen our relationships, and encourage us to pay it forward.

I have a plaque on my office wall, and I try to live by this motto daily: "Live like it's your last day." I have learned that there are no guarantees in life. Every day is a precious gift, and what we do with this gift is our choice. I hope your choice, like mine, will be to make every breath and day count.

Maintain Progress and Keep Moving Forward

Finally, I will show ways you and your family can support ongoing progress and momentum toward achieving your goals. Getting excited and diving into a new program is always easy, but it's another way to keep everyone engaged and participating. As a reminder, this program is designed to help you make lasting changes throughout your lifetime. Everyone must understand that noticeable changes will not happen on day one or in the first week. Instead, success requires heavy doses of time, patience, and consistency.

As a family unit, it will be important to remind one another of the family goals and express "high fives" for a job well done. I will discuss having weekly family talk time to discuss what is working and what is not, so that goals can be adjusted if needed. It will be essential to plan scheduled family activities throughout the week and on weekends. Additionally, at this time, the family can reflect on their progress and how far everyone has come since the program began. By being grateful for the accomplishments and hard work of the entire family, I highly encourage all my family members to share this program with their relatives and friends. I will help you understand that by helping other families in similar situations, you will continue to reinforce your success and reap greater rewards as a family.

CHAPTER 4

FAMILY TEAMWORK IS THE KEY TO SUCCESS

While growing up, my maternal grandparents, who are from China, lived with us for many years. I remember feeling so embarrassed to have these old folks at our home and refusing to have any of my friends come over. For me, the family meant eight of us in one household: my maternal grandparents, mother, father, three siblings, and me. There were always numerous chores to attend to: meals to cook, clothes to wash, and other essential daily tasks—our vegetable garden in the backyard, which my grandfather tended to with great care. We also had a variety of fruit trees, which continually supplied us with fruit throughout the year. As a young girl, all I could think of was how weird our family seemed. I always wished I could have lived in a normal American household, like the one in *Leave It to Beaver*, which I saw on TV.

Little did I know then that living in this enormous household was a blessing in disguise, as it taught me many lessons that I would later apply to my own family. My mom rarely used our clothes washer and dryer, preferring to wash clothes by hand. I was often assigned to hang the clothes on the line in our backyard and then put them away to be folded, ironed, and stored. We did have a dishwasher, but I cannot remember a single time it was ever used. I didn't have a Fitbit or pedometer back then, but I always knew I was getting plenty of daily physical activity. We had one television in our entire home. I remember looking forward to Sunday evenings, when we all gathered around to watch Walt Disney's Wonderful World of Color, followed by the TV show Bonanza, including my grandfather.

As a multigenerational family living in the same home, we were constantly together, eating, preparing meals, doing chores, watching television, and fighting. Looking back now, life seemed simple, and helping the family was necessary. As children, we never got allowances, but at the end of the day, it was nice to know that we each contributed to the family.

In today's world, technology and material possessions have overtaken us, and we are constantly using appliances such as dishwashers, washing machines, dryers, robot vacuums, remote controls for TV, and many more. Today, there is barely any need to get off our couches. No one has time for gardening, so we go to Costco and buy giant boxes of processed foods, smoothies, muffins, croissants, and other treats. Once at home, everyone microwaves their dinner and enters their rooms to eat. We even text one another, even though we are all at home and rarely have time for one-on-one conversations. We are supposed to be a family, but it feels like we're all just roommates living in the same house.

Parenting Together Consistently

Over the years, I have found that when the parents or guardians of the household can come together with clear ideas about goals or schedules and present them as a united front, the rest of the family will follow. A strong leadership team is essential for setting the direction that everyone will follow. If there are disagreements or a lack of communication between the parents or guardians, children will notice this immediately, even at an incredibly early age. As parents, we come from vastly different upbringings, values, and parenting styles. It is now essential to discuss and decide jointly with your partner on how you want to raise your children. The values and lessons we teach will hopefully lead to a happy and fulfilling life. In most cases, after these discussions, you will become clear about which direction you want to take. This process makes it easier for the entire family to be on board with the plans.

You Can Choose Your Parenting Style

I loved many aspects of my childhood, but I felt that some other elements could have been improved. As a parent, I now have a second chance to do it with my children. For example, when I was growing up, my parents never gave us many physical hugs and kisses, but I always knew they loved me. As a young parent, I discussed with my husband that I wanted our children to learn that hugging and kissing were the norm, and we agreed we would practice this daily from the time they were born. As a result, we hugged and kissed each other in front of them and gave our children abundant physical affection, which continues to feel very natural to them. This is the beauty of parents talking to one another, not making any assumptions, and moving forward as a united pair.

Rekindle the Romance

One of my favorite questions to ask my family during the office visit is, "When was the last time you went out on a date together without the children?" I will even ask this question when their child is just one month old. It is so easy to get sucked up into the overwhelming daily activities that demand your attention when you have children, especially newborns. I have seen how this soon leads to dads feeling left out and isolated. Some of the dads even get kicked out of their beds, and the child becomes the center of the entire family. As parents and family leaders, it is essential to communicate and understand each other's struggles, frustrations, and feelings. The family unit has the parents at the head and the children at the secondary. You must have these separate date nights or quiet times together to rekindle and recharge your bond as parents, which will help you see your roles more clearly. Once this is set up, parenting is much easier when you work as a team and understand who is in charge.

The children also benefit from seeing their parents spending quality time together and witnessing a successful marriage. I believe this is an incredible legacy to leave children, and they will, in turn, mimic it in their own lives as adults.

Once this hierarchy is established, with parents as the heads of the family, schedules, routines, and other family activities become much easier to enforce. The children understand that certain boundaries cannot be crossed and recognize their position within the family.

My husband and I decided early in our marriage to have "sacred" Saturday date nights. The thought of a date with my husband without children at the end of the week made my entire work week bearable. It was simple: dinner at our favorite Chinese restaurant, followed by a trip to the $1 movie theater. These quiet times were priceless and helped us connect deeper as husband and wife. I appreciated this time to recharge every weekend, be fully present with my husband, and plan for our future.

The Crucial Question for the Day

As our four children were growing up, my husband and I always had one question we asked them every evening. That question was, "What did you do for the family today?" When we came home from work, we could often hear the children scurrying around frantically putting their shoes in order, emptying the rubbish, cleaning their rooms, and so on, so that they could give us a good report. As two working parents, we had to involve the children in the household chores early on. We would always tell them that if we could finish the tasks on time, we could all go out and have some fun. Looking back, some of these free family activities were our best memories. There were activities like riding bicycles around our small community, visiting the park, or simply playing outside with the neighborhood kids.

Let's Talk about the Day

Back in the days when we were on a strict budget, my husband and I decided not to pay for cables or have an Xbox in our home. If I recall correctly, we were the last holdouts on our street for this, and our poor boys were forced to visit their neighbors to get their fill of cable TV or video games. At one point, one of our sons even looked me in the eye and asked, "Why can't we be a normal family?" I once told him we were the most normal family on our block; he did not know it yet. My husband and I often wondered if we were too strict, but you keep moving forward and do the best you can with what you have.

One of the best things we ever did as a family was gathering every evening to talk about the day before going to bed. It was a family ritual we kept going, even when the kids were in high school. We would all get together at about 8:00 p.m. after we read them books and everyone did their nighttime rituals. Everyone would have to say one thing that stood out about their day. It could be anything, and if anyone refused to contribute, they had to sit on the dreaded staircase landing "halfway up and halfway down." It was an enjoyable time of reflection on that day, and it prompted us to pause together and reflect. Most of all, it kept us informed about each other, and as I look back, it bonded us tightly as a family. It forced us to practice our communication skills and, in some cases, even made it easier to address more challenging topics later. During these nighttime talks as a family, we would take this opportunity to make special announcements of any significant changes coming up or other essential schedule changes. If my husband and I wanted input from the children, we would ask for their opinions, but they always knew that we would only take their ideas under advisement, as we would have the final say.

Be Kind to the People You Love

Family members are the people you love the most, but you sometimes forget your manners with them and occasionally fail to speak lovingly. This was something I had to work on often at home. As a pediatrician, I would listen to crying and screaming children all day, and then come home to my four young, active children, only to see chaos in the house. Before I could put my briefcase down, all four children would run to me, craving my attention. I would have a thousand things in my head to do, and start shouting out to them about what had not yet been done. There came a point where no one heard or saw me, as if I were invisible. When Dad came home later, he was greeted much more warmly. He sat down, looked them in the face, and listened to them. Finally, after much observation, I realized I needed to put my briefcase down, spend those first five minutes talking to the kids who had missed me all day, and explain to them what the plans were for the next hour and my expectations for them. At the same time, I had to be deliberately aware of how I was speaking to or treating them, just as I would with my patients and their parents throughout the day. By being kinder and acting more lovingly, I got their cooperation. Kids want to know that you love them.

I learned the hard way that our children want to know we care for them, and if we give them even five minutes of undivided attention, they will be happy and satisfied. When they were younger, we had an annual Easter tradition of hosting an Easter hunt in our backyard. The eggs each had little presents, such as candy, coins, or promissory notes, offering five or ten minutes with Mom or Dad. One Easter, I overheard the kids trying to trade their candies or coins for the notes that promised five or ten minutes with Mom or Dad, and I saw at once that they cherished the time they had with us more than material things.

Everyone Benefits from Family Connectedness

As we continue to move forward in life as a family, whenever we want to make alterations or corrections along the way, it is crucial to establish the family as the central unit and have the parents serve as the definitive leaders. The alignment of the adults in charge makes it so much easier for everyone in the family to follow along without any hesitation. This process should begin when the children are infants, but it is never too late. As families succeed in getting the children's buy-in, this same behavior follows the children in daycare and school. Respect, obedience, and teamwork that children learn at home become a pattern for them outside the house. They know their place and their boundaries and will follow the instructions given to them. Life becomes so much easier for them at home and in school, and the rewards of working together as a team become a lifelong habit. As parents, one of the greatest gifts we can give our children is the knowledge that they are valued in a loving family. Teach them self-control and respect for others. Model a devoted marriage so that they choose their partners based on this ingrained knowledge. This is how they grow strong enough to take on the challenges of adult life.

CHAPTER 5

NOURISHING OUR BODIES DAILY

Life Is Full of Decisions

There is no way around this fact—we all need to eat and nourish our bodies daily. We make decisions all day long about what to eat, when to eat, and how much to put in our mouths. This may be a conscious or unconscious decision resulting from decades of learning.

From my early childhood, I recall many memories of going into the backyard and picking the vegetables we would have for dinner in the evening. We would have green beans, bitter melon, squash, and herbs like green onions. For fruits, we would pick whatever was in season for that month and have that over and over till it was all gone from the tree.

In our modern, fast-paced world, we no longer have the luxury of time to grow, prepare, and cook together. When my children were growing up, we would go to the nearby Costco for our weekly shopping trip. Having four hungry mouths to feed always presented a challenge, especially when they came along for the shopping experience. I recall grabbing those twelve-pack muffins, croissants, and maybe even a large tub of ice cream or chips to satisfy their unending appetites. Of course, we would also ensure that we got bread, milk, fruits, and meats for the rest of the meals, but some of those other treats were so inexpensive that you couldn't resist them at the price.

In our media-savvy world, there is an overwhelming amount of information about what you should or should not eat. It is even confusing for physicians to keep up with the latest research. Many years ago, when I was growing up, we were advised to eat margarine instead of butter. However, it is now known that margarine contains too many trans fats, and we should reconsider using butter as an alternative. No wonder figuring out what you can and cannot eat is confusing.

The one motto I have stuck with throughout my years as a mom and pediatrician is that there is no such thing as forbidden food. Every food has its place in moderation. As a first-time mom, I was extremely strict with my firstborn son. With good intentions, I did my best to keep candies and other sweets out of his reach when he was a young child. However, as he got older and entered school, this strategy backfired on me. I caught him with candy wrappers under his bed and discovered this had been happening for a while. I took a different and more relaxed approach with the other two children, which turned out to be much better. They were allowed sweets, but always in moderation. Whenever there were special occasions or holidays, such as Christmas or Halloween, they could have their treats, just on a daily basis.

My Plate

Many years ago, we all followed the famous "Food Pyramid" recommendations for healthy eating. The older pyramid, introduced in 1991, was intended to serve as a nutrition guide for everyone. However, it wasn't very clear and not particularly helpful for meal planning among the general population. In May 2011, this Pyramid was replaced by the new MyPlate.

The significant difference between these two models was that grains were less emphasized. The MyPlate version reserves only one-fourth of the plate for whole grains, one-fourth of the plate for protein, and the remaining half of the plate focuses on vegetables and fruits. The MyPlate model does not specify the number of servings you should eat in any food group. If you eat from a normal-sized nine-inch plate and don't pile your food too high, you'll consume a healthy amount, promoting good weight management. This at least gives you a framework and goal to work toward. It also makes you aware of the importance of consuming fruits and vegetables.

Since we must eat daily, it is essential to understand that we must do our best to obtain all the required nutrients, including both macronutrients and micronutrients, for optimal health. Our foods can be further analyzed and classified based on their composition. Food labels now help us break down these foods and list the macronutrients and micronutrients so that we know exactly what we are about to consume. First, macronutrients provide us with calories or energy that our bodies need throughout the day. They are categorized into three groups: carbohydrates (4 calories per gram), fats (9 calories per gram), and proteins (4 calories per gram). Second, micronutrients are the substances we consume in trace amounts that our bodies need to function; unlike macronutrients, they do not provide us with any energy. Micronutrients are commonly known as vitamins and minerals that foods can be provided. Various health conditions and specific diets can lead to deficiencies in micronutrients.

The Dilemma of Picky Eaters

Many families I work with often tell me their children hate vegetables. They have tried a particular vegetable twice or thrice, and their child refuses each time.

However, I emphasize the "try a bite rule," where a specific food must sometimes be tried seven to ten times before a child develops a liking for it. I have seen this work in my patients and my children. It is also important to note that parents and other adults should be good role models and follow this rule. I tell parents to allow their child to use all their senses when trying something new. For example, they can use their fingers to feel its texture, their nose to smell it, their lips and tongue to taste it, and finally, a small bite with their teeth. If they want to spit it out, they have that right, but not in a big, dramatic way. Before moving on, their efforts to try new foods or those they dislike should be acknowledged, not praised or exaggerated.

Another unbelievably valuable concept I tell parents to put up in their kitchen is the following rule:

Parents Decide:

- What food is served
- When the food is served
- Children Decide:
- Whether or not to eat
- How much to eat

Remembering this will make mealtimes so much simpler. Both the parents and children are clear on what is expected at mealtimes. No more shouting, scolding, or negotiating ...it is what it is, and this is how it will always be. Believe it or not, this rule will help picky eaters eat better. Try it!

Take It or Leave It Rule

When our four children were growing up, I had a sign I found that read, "You have two choices for your meal today: 'Take it or leave it.'" I grew up with this rule, I was determined not to be a short-order chef, making separate meals for each family member, and my children knew it. If one of them chose not to eat, they could excuse themselves, but they were not allowed to have their meal reheated or any additional snacks or milk. They could only have water until the next meal. If that meant going to sleep hungry, then so be it, but I tell the families I work with that in all my years of practice, I have not lost a single child to starvation after skipping one meal or snack. Once the children understand the rules, they will realize the importance of eating what is presented. Thus, the benefit of being firm and consistent in this manner is that it teaches your children, especially at a young age, to eat what everyone else is eating. Ultimately, they will grow up to be great eaters as adults. This is the solution for a picky eater, but if it's not implemented early on, you'll encounter significant pushbacks. Once again, the entire family, including the caregivers, must be on board with this rule; otherwise, it will not be effective.

A final note on praising children when they eat their meal or snack. Be careful about offering excessive praise simply for eating their meals. Your children will see your response and feel more inclined to continue eating, even if they feel satisfied, to please you. Over the years, I have seen this strategy backfire, and many of these children go on to become overweight or obese adults. They continue to overeat, as this was learned in childhood, and habits, whether good or bad, are always challenging to break.

5210 Mantra

The second important concept I would like to discuss is known as the 5210 rules. This compilation of numerous rules for a healthy lifestyle has been created by health experts worldwide. After much discussion and debate, it was narrowed down to the following:

- Five servings of vegetables, roots, or fruits.
- Two hours or less of screen time per day
- One hour of physical activity daily
- Zero sugar-sweetened beverages

This easy-to-understand concept has been adapted across our nation and applies to all ages. In Hawaii, we have adopted this program and have called it the "Hawaii 5210, Let's Go Program". As a member of the Hawaii 5210 Board, I have worked over the years to disseminate this message to our entire state, including the outer islands. We have distributed posters and flyers in schools, after-school programs, YMCAs, YWCAs, sports programs, physician offices, community colleges, and other programs that touch our youth. The goal is to present a unified message on what constitutes good health throughout our entire state and help our families approach healthy living in a simplified manner. If everyone can learn, understand, and make changes whenever possible, these 5210 programs will achieve their purpose.

When reviewing the 5210 information, one question that consistently arises during our workshop sessions is, "What is a serving size?" Of course, their plates should be smaller for very young children, and servings should be given according to their size. However, for many of us, the following guidelines will also help:

- One serving of vegetables: one cup of raw or half a cup of cooked vegetables.
- One serving of fruit: half a cup of cut-up or one medium-sized fruit, about the size of a tennis ball.
- One serving of meat protein: two palm-size servings per day.
- One serving of a snack is one handful of nuts, small candies, or two handfuls of chips or pretzels.

The Hazards of Sugar-Sweetened Beverages

The one topic that is of crucial importance when it comes to the obesity crisis today is the ever-present presence of sugar-sweetened beverages. The 5210 rules state that zero to very few sugar-sweetened drinks should be consumed. As Costco shoppers, many families buy gallons of fruit punch, 100 percent orange juice, or crates of sodas, Gatorade, sweetened iced tea, Capri Sun packets, and energy drinks. We always thought fresh-squeezed orange or apple juice was healthy for many years. The reality is that one cup of concentrated fruit juice contains a high concentration of sugar, equivalent to the amount found in a can of soda. One cup of orange juice contains a sugar level equivalent to five to six oranges; drinking one or two cups of this will provide a tremendous amount of sugar in just a few minutes. Now, I can contrast this to eating five oranges in one sitting, which is virtually impossible to do. First, peeling them would take too long, and then eating five whole oranges would fill you up due to all the healthy fiber. I have always advised saving money and eating whole fruit instead of buying juices. If you love 100 percent fruit juices, then, serve this occasionally, but no more than half a cup or four ounces a day. Another trick is to dilute half of your cup of juice with water.

Again, the habits and tastes we develop in our children and ourselves will gradually take hold. After cutting back on sugar-sweetened beverages, you will likely find that they are too sweet, and water or milk will become your preferred choice. I encourage everyone to be knowledgeable about their daily drinks, as these sugar-sweetened beverages alone can lead to a lifetime of steady weight gain. I have no issue with having one or two of these drinks on weekends or for special occasions. We must know that we cannot have these daily and always think of "moderation."

Recently, at one of my family workshops, one of my dads lost five pounds in five weeks just by eliminating the one or two sodas he drank daily. If you can eliminate one can of soda a day, it is predicted that you will lose fifteen pounds a year if you do nothing else. Now, that is something to think about.

Be cautious with artificial sweeteners. There have been studies showing that people who often drink artificially sweetened drinks, such as diet sodas, end up gaining more weight than those who do not use these. This is because artificial sweeteners trick our brains into thinking we are hungry, thus causing us to eat more throughout the day. Once again, I am reminded of my initial motto of moderation in your eating and drinking habits. When I go out for dinner on the weekends, I love a weekly can of soda or orange juice; I feel I can reward myself for being so good throughout the entire week. This satisfies my cravings, and I look forward to having a sugar-sweetened beverage the following weekend.

A Word on Smoothies

Smoothies have gained considerable popularity recently, and many families I work with are incorporating them into their diets more frequently. Some families even have smoothies as part of their daily morning meals. The trouble with smoothies is that you are getting more calories and sugar when you drink a smoothie rather than eating whole fruits or vegetables. Even if you make a smoothie at home, using only fruits and vegetables, you can drink it in a few minutes, compared with the fifteen or twenty minutes it would take to eat the same number of fruits and vegetables whole. And if you're drinking smoothies frequently, you probably consume much more fruit than you would otherwise. Even though smoothies contain fiber, this fiber is broken down during the blending process, resulting in a thick paste from the fruit. Thus, you are missing out on the benefits of fiber. Fiber comes from plants and cannot be broken or absorbed by your digestive tract. It helps keep you regular, lowers cholesterol, stabilizes blood sugar levels, facilitates weight loss, and may even contribute to a longer lifespan. As a result of pulverizing the fiber in the fruits and vegetables in your smoothie, you are likely to feel hungrier soon after drinking it than you would have if you had eaten the same number of fruits and vegetables alone.

I feel it is essential for children to learn early on what each fruit or vegetable tastes, smells, and feels like, rather than simply blending it into one drink. Also, beware of commercially made or store-bought smoothies, as they often contain added sugar, honey, or other sweeteners. There is a fine line between a smoothie and a milkshake. Remember, just because it includes a leafy green, it doesn't mean it's low in calories. The bottom line is that you want smoothies to boost your nutrition, but avoid using or overusing them as a meal replacement.

Importance of Water and Milk

So, what can you drink? There are two fluids for all ages: water and milk. Calcium is an essential component of a healthy diet for all ages. Cow's milk would be the first choice, as one cup has approximately 300 milligrams of calcium per eight-ounce cup. As children grow and enter their crucial teenage years, it is recommended that they consume approximately 1,000 to 1,200 milligrams of calcium daily, in addition to adequate water intake. Studies show less than 15 percent of our teens get adequate calcium daily. Additionally, I remind parents that we, as adults, should consume milk and obtain our daily calcium intake of approximately 1,000 milligrams a day, or about two to three cups, to prevent osteoporosis and maintain our current bone mass. Once again, the adults in the house need to be good role models.

My current recommendation is that everyone two years of age and older drink skim milk, which is zero percent fat. Regular whole milk is recommended for children aged 1 to 2 years, as they require extra fat for their critical brain development.

Another interesting fact I want to share with you when deciding which cow's milk to buy is the following:

- One cup of whole milk (3 percent fat) equals the fat of eight strips of bacon.
- One cup of 2 percent milk is equal to the fat of four strips of bacon
- One cup of 1 percent milk is equal to the fat of two strips of bacon
- Finally, one cup of non-fat or skim milk has no fat.

Currently, cow milk is the preferred choice. If you are lactose intolerant, consider opting for a plant-based milk alternative. Studies are still pending on plant-based milk, as some may not contain all the nutrients found in regular cow's milk. This is where reading labels is essential to understanding what you are getting before you make a purchase.

Reading Food Labels

Learning how to read food labels is an important skill when shopping. Whenever looking at food labels, it is essential to first scan the serving size. For example, one twenty-four-ounce can of Arizona Green Tea contains approximately thirteen tablespoons of sugar. If you read the food label carefully, you will see that this product can come in three serving sizes. Thus, one serving of this beverage would comprise approximately eight ounces (or one-third of the contents of the entire can). If you're like most people who drink this beverage, you likely finish the whole can in one sitting.

Another effective label-reading practice is checking the sugar content in breakfast cereals. Always look at the serving sizes and then the sugar content. Generally, if a cereal has over 14 grams of sugar per serving, it is likely too sweet. Through my workshops, many families I work with, including the children, learn to become label readers and more informed consumers. I encourage families to shop and examine food labels for the best value. This can be a game changer in improving overall health choices. For myself, I used to buy many preprocessed ready-to-eat frozen foods from Costco in bulk, but after reading Food labels, which display the amount of fat and sodium in these foods, have altered my purchasing habits. It is always best to stick with simple, whole foods and prepare them in your kitchen, without all the added preservatives and chemicals.

My final advice is to choose foods lower in fat, cholesterol, sodium, and sugar. Instead, look for foods higher in fiber, vitamins, minerals, and protein. As discussed earlier in this chapter, micronutrients (vitamins and minerals) and fiber are essential for daily bodily functions. Your body will thank you for your wiser choices.

Meal Prep as a Family

Sit down as a family and discuss the available food options. Check out the weekly food and specials to buy items that are in season or on sale. Based on this, plan your menu around these foods and take the entire family to shop with your list. Shopping at the farmers' market can sometimes be more affordable, as it eliminates the middleman and cuts out the middleman, going directly from farm to table. Consider checking it out on weekends as a family activity. I also like Costco as an alternative to fresh fruits and vegetables, as it offers a wide range of produce in its freezer section. I often enjoy the convenience of the small frozen Birdseye vegetable boxes that can be placed in the microwave and on the table in just a few minutes.

If they are old enough, get the children to wash and help prepare the fruits and vegetables, or participate in the cooking. This gets everyone excited about the final product and more likely to eat the masterpiece they have helped create.

Another excellent family idea is starting a vegetable garden at home. It could be as simple as getting a five-gallon plastic tub and planting a tomato plant or herbs. The excitement of harvesting the first tomato, washing it, and then eating it is indescribable. The children become so connected to the earth, their plants, and the fruit of their labor that they become eager for more.

Think outside the Box

One of the questions I heard daily from my family was, "What's for dinner, Mom?"

When feeding my family many years ago, I quickly discovered that everyone loved their meat. When my teenage boys came home after school, I would have to label the container with beef with an extensive sign reading, "This is for dinner – do not eat this." Thus, there were many meals when I would serve everyone their portion of meat, and other choices on the table could supplement the rest of the meal. I always liked having a green tossed salad, brown rice, stir-fried vegetables, frozen vegetables, and fruit served. Additionally, I loved making large pots of hearty homemade soups to offer as appetizers or serve with meals.

For breakfast, I did not limit our menu to traditional "breakfast foods." Instead, I would pull out leftovers from the night before and offer more of these vegetables and fruits. If there were leftovers from breakfast, the remainder would be packed up for lunch. I continue to practice this daily with my lunch. My staff teases me that I'm the "Tupperware Queen" of portion control, and they always want to see the assortment of food I'm having for lunch. For me, the best part of my workday is lunch.

I must admit that, as a busy young mother, there were days when I had to resort to buying from fast-food establishments or ordering takeout from restaurants. I will get your basic burgers, chicken tenders, pizza, or entrée and bring them home. I would supplement this meal with lettuce salad, tomatoes, cheese, milk, water, and fruits. In Hawaii, we have plate lunches consisting of protein, two scoops of white rice, and macaroni. If I brought these plate lunches home, I would supplement this meal with fruits, veggies, water, and milk. One of my favorite ways to stretch a dinner meal was to go to Panda Express, pick up combo plates or the "Family Feast," and then take it home to add more vegetables to the stir-fried entrées. For example, I would stir-fry fresh broccoli in the beef broccoli entrée, and many times, no additional seasoning was needed. Everyone would get their vegetables for dinner, but my kids always knew what I did and would roll their eyes.

For each family, figure out what works for you. Sit down as a family to discuss the many options for healthier choices that get everyone excited and start at this point. I guarantee it will slowly snowball into other exciting projects and significant decisions.

CHAPTER 6

MOVE MORE

Kids Are No Longer "Free Range"

Growing up in Hawaii, where the weather is consistently sunny and 80 degrees year-round, with only occasional light showers, made it easy to want to be outdoors all the time. Of course, those good old days were days of innocence – once we completed our household chores, our parents forced my siblings and me to play outside until dinner time. We had so much fun outdoors with the neighborhood kids, playing with cardboard boxes, searching for earthworms, and simply roller-skating up and down the street without a care in the world. I do not recall any twenty-four-hour fitness gyms, Curves, or other exercise facilities back then. The only exercise class I ever saw as a child was the *Jack LaLanne Show* on the few television channels we had at the time. I remember following along and listening to his health tips. I especially loved seeing his lovely wife, Elaine, come in to help.

For me, exercise was moving around and doing it daily without even thinking about it. I did not have PE in elementary or middle school, but we always had recess and lunch, where I loved to play tetherball or volleyball or just run around like a crazy person until sweat was streaming down the side of my face. Now, that was a great workout!

Now, let's go forward to today. As a mother of four young children, I rarely allow them to play outdoors alone. I recall reading a very popular book called "Don't Talk to Strangers." Back in the eighties, there was a young boy named Adam Walsh who was kidnapped from Sears and then found murdered. Many more horror stories kept coming up, like Ted Bundy, the serial killer, and finally, we had the tragedy of September 11, 2001. I remember it was Tuesday morning in Hawaii, and our entire family watched the live broadcast in disbelief as the second tower fell. Thus, in this new and modern, ever-changing world, my children were rarely allowed to be "free range" as I had many things to do once I got home and did not have the time and energy to be outside supervising them. As they got older, it was always a struggle for more freedom, but again, I always felt like I had to have a tight rein on them, considering the world as it is today.

Self-Care Tossed Aside

Caring for myself seemed like a luxury I could not afford while raising the kids and working full-time. I had neither money nor time for gym membership. In my younger, single days, I loved to jog, swim, or play tennis as much as possible. I considered working out while cleaning the kitchen, showers, and toilets, sweeping, cooking, grocery shopping, raking leaves, and all the other things mothers do. At the office, I was on my feet constantly, jumping from room to room to see my patients and frequently wrestling with them to administer their shots. Throughout all of this, I felt very resentful for having to do it all and felt like I never had a good attitude about this. Looking back, it was an extremely stressful time in my life, and it was just a matter of survival from day to day.

A New Perspective

As I mentioned earlier, this stress culminated in a significant depression for me at the age of forty. I never thought this could happen to me, but it did, and I am grateful as I look back on this time. I knew I had to reset my priorities and accept help from my husband, children, parents, and in-laws. For a few years, my husband even included a budget for a housekeeper to come twice a month to help with the cleaning.

With a new and better outlook on chores, I began to see how we could all have specifically assigned chores and accomplish things together more efficiently. The children were assigned to keep their rooms clean and tidy, clean the bathroom, fold their clothes, set the table, help with dishes, and perform other tasks to support the family.

Working with a psychiatrist, I began to feel myself again and see things in a new light. This realization changed how I viewed many things, including even the mundane tasks like household chores. With the entire family chipping in and helping, I suddenly saw chores as an opportunity for family time and accomplishing things together in a shorter period. Once tasks were completed, knowing this was a team effort felt good. One of the things we would do as a family, after completing our chores on the weekend, was reward ourselves with an outdoor family outing to one of the many beautiful parks, beaches, or trails in Hawaii.

The Family That Works Together Plays Together

As the children grew older, it became a tradition to do chores together over the weekend and then discuss where we would go. Back in the "old" days, there were few soccer, baseball, or flag football sports groups, so my husband and I would devise our family activities.

Looking back, these simple activities were among the best family times and memories I can recall. All six of us would go bicycling or take after-dinner walks around the neighborhood. We would often have weekend picnics at the beach or enjoy the neighborhood parks, complete with jungle gyms, monkey bars, and other play equipment. The kids were always the happiest when they were outdoors with us, and I know that money could not buy this.

There were times when I thought I had too many things to do at home, but I forced myself to go out with the family, and I have never regretted a minute of it. I always heard my elders telling me to enjoy my young children because they will all be grown up before you know it. I could never believe this statement because when caring for four young children, all you can think is, "When are you going to grow up and do things for yourself?" My advice is to believe it when people tell you to cherish your children when they're young, because it's true. In the blink of an eye, they graduate from high school and perhaps college, get married, and start their own families.

Cub Scouts and Boy Scouts

An excellent activity that entered our lives when our three boys were younger was the Cub Scouts of America and the Boy Scouts of America. Our neighbors started this in our young neighborhood, and we finally joined them. This was one of the best things we ever did for our boys. We had weekly Cub Scout meetings at our home where they would learn how to cook, tie knots, and much more. We would have overnight camp-overs in our backyard. Even our daughter, the youngest in the family, took part in the activities we had at our home. As the boys advanced into Boy Scouts, we continued the planned family activities once a month and even assisted each boy with their Eagle Projects. Now that my children are grown up and have families, we have wonderful memories of time spent together. My children never once talked about the material possessions they had, but fondly recalled the time we spent together doing things as a family. I genuinely believe that this is an ongoing issue.

Connectivity builds daily and helps us develop a genuine bond that keeps us happy and fulfilled in good times and bad.

Dancing Together as a Family

My youngest daughter also had an activity outlet: dancing. She began lessons at the age of three under the tutelage of sixteen-year-old teacher Wendy Calio at Sabrina Starr Dance Studios in Wahiawa. Stephen and I both had office hours on Saturday mornings, so we had to enroll her in something that would keep her busy on Saturdays. Fortunately, she enjoyed and thrived in dancing, and she soon brought the passion of dancing into the home.

At home, we would start "free dancing" to random music and not even know why we were doing it. When movement is done as a spontaneous activity, it doesn't feel like exercise, but rather like something to share. I recall one incident where I heard Christmas music, and I got so excited that I started dancing, spinning, and then tripped out of control, knocking over a nearby table. We might have even had that on video, but I remember laughing hard and having fun doing "free dance."

As the children grew older, they wanted to go to the gym in high school, but I could not see us spending money on that. With four healthy children, I instead asked them to consider doing extra household chores as their exercise, like car washing, yard work, and additional cleaning. When our boys were older in high school, we had them take on summer jobs at the school, such as helping the janitor or assisting with landscaping, to gain real-life experience. This time, we accomplished something. I heard some complaining, but overall, it made them more capable adults and helped them learn to appreciate the value of money and the little things more.

Activities in our family just seemed to evolve naturally as a way of life. We even recruited the boys to participate in their sisters' dance activities, such as participating in The Nutcracker or helping make decorations for various parades and recitals. The four children loved their sports and participated in volleyball and basketball. They may not have been the most outstanding players, but they sure had fun, and I thoroughly enjoyed attending their games to cheer them on. My third son enjoyed being a rebel, and instead of joining the school sports, he became a wonderful skateboarder. This love of movement and activities has continued regularly throughout their lives, even during their college years and as young adults. As their mother, it's terrific to see that exercise is viewed as something enjoyable, and they continue to incorporate it into their daily routines.

The Very Best Exercise for Everyone

As I age and become more tech-savvy, a wrist pedometer is one of the best devices I've recently bought. It's not a fancy Fitbit, but I saw it online for $30. This was the best investment I have ever made, and it even records my blood pressure, heart rate, and pulse. Since I am naturally competitive, I now track my daily steps to maximize them. It has motivated me to challenge myself and others and reminds me to keep walking throughout the day. When I park far away from my destination, I feel thrilled to be able to take more steps, especially if I have been sitting in front of my computer all day. If I shop after work, especially at large stores like Costco, I love walking up and down the aisles for more steps.

It has been commonly noted that 10,000 steps a day is a reasonable estimate for adults to take each day to achieve good health. However, in a recent study examining nearly 17,000 women, scientists found that the sweet spot for reducing the risk of premature death by 40 percent was 4,500 steps per day. Women who moved more definitely had fewer premature deaths, up to a plateau of about 7,500 steps a day. So, with my family participants, I always encourage them to count their steps and know that taking more steps is better than taking fewer.

Research has consistently shown that walking is the most effective exercise for people of all ages. No equipment is needed; it is accessible anytime, and there is a minimal risk of injury. As a result, walking has the lowest dropout rate, and the benefits are numerous.

Walk with a Doc – Oahu

With this information in mind, I decided to start my local chapter of the Walk with a Doc nonprofit organization called Walk with a Doc – Oahu. My mentor, colleague, and later dear friend, Dr. Annemarie Sommer, was a renowned geneticist. She was one of the original, staunch advocates of this now worldwide program. After several years of encouragement and nudging from her, I finally decided it was time to bring it to my island of Oahu. My fellow medical school Classmate Dr. Craig Kadooka had already started a Walk with a Doc group in Hilo on the Big Island of Hawaii, which had met with much success, so it was time to bring it to Oahu! As you may recall, I initiated my free weekly community event, Walk with a Doc—Oahu, in my community, where people of all ages and fitness levels could come together and walk with me in a non-traditional setting.

I loved this worldwide program from the moment I heard about it. The mastermind behind this movement is Dr. David Sabgir, a cardiologist in Columbus, Ohio, who initiated this revolutionary program approximately fifteen years ago. He thought outside the box and asked his patients to improve their health by walking with him on a Saturday at the nearby park. This idea took off like wildfire, and soon, walking groups began to emerge all over the United States, then spreading to other countries. It is now in over twenty-five countries with more than five hundred walking groups worldwide.

I began my Walk with a Doc – Oahu group in February 2016, and we are now entering our tenth year of offering this free weekly program at nearby Patsy T. Mink – Central Oahu Regional Park on Saturdays from 8:00 to 9:00 AM. Walkers range in age from one to ninety-four. I know that much of the success of my weekly program is due to the fellowship and support we provide each week, which helps us strive for good health. Just getting their shoes on and driving out at 8:00 a.m. on Saturday means commitment, and

I will always acknowledge that. There are so many times when I wake up on Saturday morning thinking of every excuse in the book not to go, but I do it for them. After all, I am Doc! Once it's done, I feel so proud of myself for the effort, and it's a great way to start the weekend! My walkers think I am helping them, but they are the ones who are motivating me to get out there and exercise.

Hike with a Doc and Dance with a Doc

Additionally, since most of my walkers are fifty and older, I have received numerous requests to participate in activities beyond just Walking with a Doc. In response to their requests, I initiated a new supplemental program called Hike with a Doc, which follows immediately after our Walk with a Doc program. From May to September, our seniors and other walkers enjoy exploring nearby walking paths and routes. This proved to be a very popular and enjoyable addition since hiking together in a group is always more fun.

Due to the sometimes-rainy weather during winter and spring, I stopped the Hike with a Doc program and replaced it with Dance with a Doc, Cook with a Doc, or Craft with a Doc. These activities have become a smash hit, and everyone enjoys the additional opportunities to get to know one another and share their stories. At each event, we gather for a potluck, and everyone brings their favorite dish to share. This fellowship time together solidifies our community as a "walking family." It reinforces that we are not alone and have a common goal to live in optimal health for years to come.

Moving More Daily – A Lifelong Goal

Incorporating movement into your life must be a lifelong pursuit that involves creativity, purposeful intent, and fun. I have found that when activity incorporates family and friends, it is something that most of us can maintain for a lifetime. So, I now challenge you to step out and find a happy place with movement. Be daring and try a new sport or join others in activities like water aerobics, yoga, Zumba, or anything else that seems interesting to you, and reap the rewards. You will be proud of yourself and your family just for trying.

CHAPTER 7

THE INCREDIBLE VALUE OF SLEEP AND FAMILY MEALS

Family Mealtimes Are Crucial

Scientific studies have shown the importance of eating healthy, scheduled meals for an energy boost, improved memory, sharper focus, and better appetite control between meals. That quick snack or pick-me-upper is rarely the most nutritious choice, and it is generally something sweet and starchy. This snack will satisfy you only for a short time. When the next meal rolls by, you will realize you already had your little cheat snack, so another meal will pass. What happens to most people, especially teens, is that they become so hungry after school that they have a substantial snack or a full meal with their friends or at home. This, in turn, leads to feelings of heaviness, sluggishness, and fatigue. They will frequently feel like taking a nap, and then when dinner swings by, it will not interest them. They will hit the refrigerator for a late-night snack when hunger strikes again in the early evening.

This same pattern seems to occur for many adults as well. Thus, I have seen many first-year college students gain the infamous "Freshman fifteen," or a weight gain of fifteen pounds, after their first year of college time and time again.

Increasingly, studies confirm that eating meals together as a family has numerous benefits. Often, this is the only time when all family members are together in one place. Family meals can seem like a burden at the end of a tiring day, but the many benefits will be worth the extra effort. Eating together promotes more sensible eating habits, which in turn helps everyone manage their weight better. When families sit together, a special bond develops over time, allowing each member to better cope with life's daily stresses.

Children need to know that parents and siblings are there to listen to and support each other. The conversation over the dinner table can be as simple as "How was your day?" or "What was the best thing that happened to you today?" By listening to what your children say, you are saying, "I value what you do; I respect who you are and what you are doing;

what you do is important to me." Mealtimes should be viewed as an opportunity with all kinds of possibilities. Parents can help their children learn valuable lessons, such as good table manners, practical communication skills, and the importance of listening and respecting one another. It is also an ideal way to review the day and plan for the next day.

Sleep Is Learned Behavior

So, let's back up and see how we can avoid this situation. The number one excuse I hear from my patients for not eating breakfast is that they are too tired. My quick response to this is, "Go to bed earlier." This is easier said than done. When discussing breakfast, we must also consider sleep, as these two factors are closely intertwined. Both sleep and family meals are crucial factors in helping people of all ages manage their weight and perform at their best the next day.

In our modern world, sleep has developed a bad reputation and become something we often put at the bottom of our list of priorities. I occasionally hear my colleagues bragging about how little sleep they get, and they think that they can still perform well. However, the truth is that sleep is essential for total body restoration, muscle repair, immune system improvement, enhanced memory storage, and overall well-being. Numerous studies have been conducted on the importance of sleep, and it is undeniable that its significance is substantial. If you are not getting enough sleep, you rob your body of something vital to thrive.

Developing sound and consistent sleep habits is crucial for all ages, particularly for young individuals. From the first time I saw newborn babies in my office, I began discussing the importance of sleep for babies and chronically tired parents. The keys to developing great sleep habits are consistency and continued reinforcement of your sleep rituals. What this means is that, whether it's a weekday or a weekend, everyone in the family strives to have a consistent bedtime ritual, which may include brushing and flossing teeth, reading a book, praying, discussing the day, giving a goodnight kiss, and then going to bed. After over thirty-five years of practicing as a pediatrician, I have found that for parents who heed my advice and allow this pattern to continue, their newborn babies soon learn to self-soothe and sleep eight to ten hours through the night by three to four months of age. The new parents I work with say it is impossible, but I have seen it repeatedly, and all four of my children were sleeping through the night by four months of age.

My theory is that if this works for babies, it can work for people of any age. Sleep is a learned behavior; you can always change behavior regardless of age. For the older children and teens I work with, I always tell them that everyone must understand the value of sleep and the urgency of getting the recommended hours. By forming nighttime rituals that everyone can participate in, success is more likely to occur. Again, the easiest way to do this is to set bedtimes for your kids, depending on their age, and reinforce nighttime rituals, such as reading or discussing the day as a family. Additionally, try to turn off all electronics at least 30 minutes to one hour before bedtime. The rest of the family will follow if the adults are all in. The teens will know if the parents are all in by observing their behavior, so you will develop their trust by following along. I guarantee that once the family sleeps better, everyone will feel much better, and the likelihood of eating breakfast will increase.

Sleep Recommendation

The following are the recommended hours of sleep by the National Sleep Foundation according to age, but remember, everyone's sleep needs are different:

- Ages three to five years: eleven to thirteen hours
- Ages five to twelve years: ten to eleven hours
- Adolescents: eight and a half to nine and a half hours
- Adults: seven to nine hours

Power Naps

A question I often get is about the value of naps. It is essential to avoid taking long afternoon naps, as this may leave one too awake to fall asleep at night. Instead of long naps of over two to three hours during the day, if you or your child needs to recharge your batteries, try a "power nap." Power naps are designed to revitalize oneself from drowsiness and should be limited to twenty to thirty minutes in duration. These naps should also occur before 4:00 p.m. to avoid disrupting nighttime sleep schedules.

By getting adequate sleep at night, everyone will be more easily able to wake up in a better mood, feel better, and avoid the foggy daytime sleepiness that can last all day. Adequate sleep will help you boost your metabolism, feel more energized to be active, and have a reduced tendency to eat sweet, starchy foods throughout the day. The bottom line is that getting enough sleep helps control your weight and so much more.

Be Careful about Screen Time

On another note, as we discussed sleep earlier, I mentioned that screen time is now one of the greatest sleep robbers. It is crucial to remove all the screens from your children's bedrooms to eliminate temptation. The bedroom should be associated with rest and sleep; without the screens of television or iPads, sleep becomes much easier. Again, parents must also heed this advice and consider the same for themselves. Recent studies have shown that the "blue light" emitted by our screens can harm sleep. As a pediatrician, one of the first things I tell young parents is not to use the television or iPad as a substitute for supervision. The American Academy of Pediatrics recommends limiting screen time to zero for children under the age of three. This even includes Sesame Street and the PBS television station. Studies show that screen time does not stimulate the young mind, and, in fact, just talking, reading, and interacting with your young child will be far more beneficial in helping to develop good habits for your child later in life. Thus, I recommend that no television, video games, or other similar electronics be used in any bedroom from the beginning to promote sleep and overall better health habits.

Importance of Preplanning Meals and Snacks

Preplanning is one of the keys to eating breakfast daily or preparing home lunches. In the morning, I admit I'm still a bit foggy, but I've already planned what I want to eat the night before. With my young children, whenever I picked them up from school or after an event, I always had a cooler of fruits, veggies, and water ready for them. Not only did they enjoy a good snack, but they also saved a significant amount of money. Yes, we occasionally took our children to fast-food restaurants, but this was the exception.

Another great tip I used for preplanning was to use the weekend to create two or three large pots of stews, soups, or sauces for the coming week. By doing this, dinner would be ready within minutes after coming home from work. Another quick solution was using my crockpot for a great, ready-to-eat hot dinner at the end of the day. When you're heating dinner or setting the table, this is an excellent time for the children to help you prepare their lunches and snacks for the next day. By doing this, everyone gets involved in the meal and snack preparation, and family members are more likely to eat what they have helped to prepare.

Baby Step Changes

Sleep and breakfast offer numerous benefits for everyone in the family. Consider discussing this topic with children of all ages. It's never too late for parents and grandparents to readjust their schedule. In the next chapter, we will discuss taking small, baby steps and setting goals as you move forward toward changing a lifetime of unhealthy habits. Remember, the slower the change is implemented, the more permanent it is. As I tell the families I work with, if you haven't cleaned your home in two or three years, don't expect to complete the job in two or three weeks. Investing time and effort to make healthy changes will multiply the rewards you reap for years.

CHAPTER 8

SMALL GOALS AMOUNT TO BIG WINS

When I was a young girl, my dad had a weekly tradition of taking all four of us to the main public library on Friday nights to borrow books. This was the highlight of my week, as my dad worked on weeknights from Monday through Thursday. I loved to read biographies of famous people. I soon found myself reading the biographies of famous women, such as Florence Nightingale, Marie Curie, and Elizabeth Blackwell, the first woman to receive a medical degree in the United States. I was so fascinated by Dr. Blackwell's story that I told my family I wanted to be a woman physician at the age of seven. This was back in the 1960s, and I didn't even know of a woman doctor in Hawaii, but I thought this was what I wanted to be.

As a young child, I had no clue about goal setting, but I made it a daily goal to take a step closer each day toward that goal. For example, whenever anyone needed a bandage, I would run to get it. I would always accompany my mom to visit my grandparents or relatives who were hospitalized. Whenever I saw a physician, I would picture myself already working as a physician, complete with a stethoscope around my neck and a crisp white coat.

I wanted to begin this chapter with my story of goal setting and how my crazy dream became a reality. Later in the chapter, I will also share with you other techniques that have been shown to help many set and achieve specific goals.

Grit Makes the Difference

As a young girl who wanted to become a doctor, my family was always very encouraging, especially my father. When other people approached me and told me this was not a good idea, it gave me more fuel to prove them wrong. For many years, I remember picturing myself as an adult, wearing a white coat, having already achieved this audacious dream of becoming a woman doctor. I lived and breathed this dream daily, through my schoolwork, outside activities, and everything I did. I always knew I was not the smartest in my class, but I always worked hard. Back in my school days, the Catholic nuns gave us two grades: one for our actual work and a second for effort. I know the first column was not always A's, but the second column's grade for effort was always excellent. After a test or challenge, my dad always asked me, "Did you try your best?" I always answered yes, and he kept urging me to move forward.

The same approach also seemed to work with sports. At twelve years old, I learned how to play tennis and loved it. Within a year, I was on the Maryknoll High School tennis team, and I recall spending hours on the Ala Moana tennis court, hitting balls against the backboard, trying to perfect my serve or strokes. Playing a sport in high school taught me the valuable lesson of striving to achieve my goals and putting in hard work every day.

You Can't Force Anyone to Do Something They Don't Want to Do

Fast-forward to being a young, working mother with four active children and trying to apply these same rules to dealing with life's challenges. Yes, I had big goals for myself, my work, my family, and my children, but now I realize this is a whole new ball game. This was no longer just about me, but about the other family members as well. I quickly learned I got a lot of resistance if I forced someone to do something because I wanted it for them. An example to illustrate this point is when my third son was in elementary school, and he would bring home Cs. He was a brilliant young man, and I told him I knew he had a lot of potential, to which he immediately replied, "What's wrong with a C? I am an average person like most people." This was a hard pill to swallow, as I was not used to my children being uncertain of their potential, not working to the best of their ability, or setting goals for the future. From a young age, I always thought everyone knew their purpose in life and how to achieve it. This was a big reality check for me.

Everyone Pitches In

After my severe depressive episode at age forty, my husband and I finally realized that we needed the entire family to pitch in and help with everyday chores; we divided the household chores according to age and abilities. There were daily chores, as well as weekends and monthly chores.

No allowance was offered for this, and our children were repeatedly told in our home that this is just what a family does and that this was their way of contributing to the family.

With consistency, reminders, and time, the kids slowly accepted their responsibilities and completed the assigned tasks. I think it made them feel proud to do their part for the family and learn life skills that would be very helpful as they started living independently.

Setting goals as a family, especially with younger children, has always been challenging. My husband and I did not have a book or outline to follow back then, but I did want to share with you an approach that seemed to work very well for the families I worked with in our recent family workshops. This approach has been employed by many over the years in various situations and has yielded considerable success.

Goal Setting Method

This method is called the S.M.A.R.T. approach.

- **S = specific:** What exactly do you want to achieve?
- **M=measurable:** How will you know you have completed it?
- **A= attainable:** Is it something you can control?
- **R= relevant:** Why is this applicable to your life?
- **T= time-based:** How long will it take to achieve your goals?

Families or individuals can use this method to write down a specific goal. The following is an example of a vague goal that would not work well: "I want our family to get healthier." The discussion should be more specific, like "Our family will walk together for at least fifteen minutes every day for the next two weeks." This goal is doable and achievable for the entire family. It is a way to form a healthy habit, and the chances of success are greater with everyone buying in.

Additionally, if adults want to set individual goals, these could be implemented in conjunction with family goals. For example, if the parents want to sneak in fifteen minutes of walking after dinner, this could be piggybacked with the family goal of increasing overall physical activity. If other family members are free, they could also accompany Mom or Dad on this extra walk. It is always a good idea to write down the agreed-upon family goals and Place it on the refrigerator so each family member can remind one another to do this daily. Psychologists now say it takes about thirty consecutive days to make a habit permanent. It makes sense to choose a new family goal at the start of every month or at regular intervals and review how the previous goal was achieved.

Start Small and Succeed

When you and your family start setting goals, remember always to take small bites, not big ones. Succeeding in these smaller goals will boost your confidence in tackling the larger goals.

Ultimately, taking lifestyle changes to the extreme rarely proves effective. Some families tell me they want to be healthier and immediately stop eating rice or starches altogether. They start to lose weight; however, this can only last for a limited time. Soon, they return to their old eating habits, and their weight increases again. It is now established that these patterns of fluctuating weights can be more detrimental to your health, so it is advisable to make changes gradually. Remember that the more gradual the change, the more permanent the change. It will be hard work, and there will be days when you don't feel like it but keep pressing on and investing in your future success. Keep your eye on the goal and the rewards that will come.

When I was a young girl, my dad taught me a portion of a poem by Henry Wadsworth Longfellow. I recited and thought of it so many times that I committed it to my memory. I even used it as my comment under my senior photo, and it goes like this:

> *"The heights great men have achieved and kept were not attained by a single flight, But they, while their companions slept, were toiling upward through the night."*

This poem was instrumental in encouraging me to push forward on what seemed, at times, like an impossible dream: to become a woman physician back in the 1970s. Despite failures and disappointments along the way, I knew it would take hard work and perseverance to accomplish this goal. I feel blessed to have had the help of many mentors, and I now strive to pay it forward by serving as a mentor to high school, pre-med, medical students, and residents as they progress along their journeys.

CHAPTER 9

LIFE IS ABOUT BEING IN THE PRESENT MOMENT

I t is sometimes fun to look back and recall carefree childhood memories. One of the first things that came to my mind was how happy and free I felt as a young girl when I went roller-skating for hours up and down the street I lived on. I can recall the cracks in the sidewalks, the houses I passed by, and the details of my neighbors' homes and yards. Without knowing it, I savored every moment of joy that filled me, and it has always been—and will always be—my place from childhood.

As a young, busy mother, there were so many things to do that I felt like I missed being present at many moments with my kids. I was always thinking of future tasks and worrying about whether I had made the right decisions in the past. I recall looking at my youngest one day when she was four and wondering, "How did you grow up so quickly?" It is sometimes even harder for me to recall the details of my children's childhood. Despite all the mishaps and mistakes my husband and I may have made, I am happy to know they are decent human beings. The few moments I remember are when I could focus on them and enjoy that special time of being fully present with each of them.

Social media robs us of time. In today's quick-paced world, one cannot help but be caught up in all this busyness. Our social media on smartphones, tablets, computers, and other electronics constantly shows us what others are doing, the many activities available to us, and much more, all at the touch of a button. Sometimes, we spend so much time scrolling through social media that an hour passes before we decide to do something.

Practice being present 100 percent of the time. In our recent workshops with parents, I learned some practical tips for living in this so-called present moment. It has opened my eyes to a better way of living, one that brings more joy and fulfillment. I am not thinking of the past or future by focusing on my present activity. At times, I won't even take out my phone camera to take vacation photos; instead, I savor where I am, who I'm with, and what I'm feeling, taking in all that I can at that moment. This has given me a better memory. Of course, this is something new for me, and I try to practice it daily.

When I am at work and seeing patients, I take a deep breath as I touch the doorknob to open the door and try to clear my mind to be fully present for the patient. Recently, it has also helped me slow down my eating habits. Due to having a busy schedule my entire life, I realized that I had become conditioned to eat as quickly as possible. It seemed to be something I was proud of. Still, as I examined this habit, I realized it was leading to me overeating many times and not appreciating the whole eating experience. By taking the time to slow down my eating deliberately and even taking at least eight to ten bites per mouthful while putting my fork down, I can feel the texture of the food, appreciate the smell, appearance, and taste, and be fully aware of this meal. I also found that by eating this way, I could be mindful of feeling full and understand when to stop.

Help Each Other Be Mindful

Another advantage for many of our workshop participants was that they became aware of their impulses and weaknesses. An example of this is my awareness of my love of ice cream. If I know I have ice cream in my freezer, it's hard to resist it as a snack at night. A solution I came up with was not to buy a half-gallon carton in my home freezer, but instead to eat fruit or brush my teeth, call it a day, and go to bed. By understanding this, you can manage your environment so that this impulse is neither acted upon nor avoided.

Young children's brains are not yet fully developed, so they require the guidance of their parents, grandparents, or other adults to help them develop mindfulness, which can lead to better decision-making.

One of the techniques that my husband and I used with our kids for discipline was the well-known "timeout." Timeouts were used for specific reasons, such as if our child did something to hurt themselves or others; this was a definite timeout. Our child's age determines the length of timeouts. For example, if our child were ten years old, they would have to sit in the boring timeout corner for ten minutes. The rule of thumb was one minute for each year of life. Overall, we found this to be quite effective, and upon reflection, I now see that it gave our children quiet time to reflect on what had brought them there in the first place.

Meditation: The Pause Button

When my husband and I raised our four children in the 1980s and 1990s, we always had "quiet time" on Sunday afternoons, when everyone would lie down for an hour to rest and take a break. We also utilized a technique called "time-outs" whenever the children engaged in actions that could have harmed themselves or others. The whole point of these timeouts was to have the child sit in a quiet corner and reflect on what misdeed they had just committed.

The current terminology or trendy word we now use is 'meditation.' From conducting our recent family workshops, I have observed the numerous benefits that meditation offers to people of all ages. Taking even a few moments to connect with where you are or how you're feeling can help you make better decisions moving forward. If things start getting hectic at work and I fall behind in the schedule, I take a few seconds to breathe, regroup, and remind myself to be 100 percent present for every new patient I see that day. This has helped me tremendously in listening fully to patients and their parents, making the right decisions and choices. Like any new habit, this skill requires time and practice.

Practice Belly Breathing

One of the homework assignments that was very helpful for our families was choosing and practicing one of the many free meditation resources available online. One of their favorites was "belly breathing" to help calm, destress, and relax instantly. This is performed by placing a stuffed animal on your tummy, then lying down comfortably for a few minutes, and watching your belly rise and fall as you concentrate on this and nothing else. I have been doing this recently, especially when so many thoughts rush through my head at night. I start belly breathing three to four times and focus on my breathing. By doing this often, I generally find myself falling asleep immediately. The beauty of this is that almost anyone, regardless of age, can succeed.

Meditation can help you calm down and reconnect with your desire to be healthier. It can also help you focus, make better decisions, and be more disciplined. I am still new to this, but I see success in others and will continue to practice.

Once again, every person and family are unique. Try a different meditation technique if belly breathing doesn't work for you. Mindfulness and meditation can be a practice that the entire family can engage in together, and I believe it could lead to a more harmonious life.

CHAPTER 10

A POSITIVE ATTITUDE CHANGES EVERYTHING

Be Kind to Yourself and Others

The process of changing one's lifetime habits is not easy. We always strive to do our best to accomplish the goals we set, but the truth is that we are bound to make mistakes. Here is a big secret: you are human, and none of us is perfect. I hope you don't condemn yourself or others for these moments of weakness or mishaps.

For some reason, your brain tends to focus on the negatives rather than the positives. It is much easier to criticize negative behavior in ourselves or others, and it isn't easy to point out the positives when they do occur. In my mind and experience, I know this, but it's rare to pick each other up and point out times when you or others are doing something positive.

Give Praise Freely

As a pediatrician, I always give this advice to young parents. I remind them to pay close attention to their child's positive behaviors and reward them for these behaviors, rather than focusing on their negative behaviors. For example, if your child reacts positively to the new baby brought home, be sure to mention this. If you don't, your child will try to get your immediate reaction by doing something they were told not to do.

By practicing this attitude of gratitude, you will be more likely to exhibit this positive behavior. Praise or positive feedback could include: "I saw that you chose the apple instead of the Oreo cookies...good choice" or "You're right. I did not walk the dog tonight. Would you like to join me?". When we give someone positive feedback for a specific behavior, that person is more likely to repeat that behavior because of the positive feeling it evokes.

The recipient of positive praise benefits from the positive comments, but the giver of praise also benefits. Studies show that those who give positive praise are happier now, but research has also shown that this happiness continues for the giver for months to follow. By getting into the habit of writing thank-you notes or a sentence or two in a gratitude journal will make you much more aware of the good and abundance in your life. More research indicates that practicing gratitude can alter your outlook on life, enhance your sleep quality, disposition, and immune system function.

The Value of Relationships

When we talk about being grateful, it is always a good idea to teach our children to focus on the relationships they have in their lives rather than material possessions or experiences. With many millennials currently in high credit card debt, it's essential to prioritize what is most important in our lives, and ultimately, these are the close relationships we have formed over the years.

As our young children grew up, my husband and I struggled financially while growing our private practices. We decided not to buy brand-name shoes or clothes for ourselves and the children, and we held out for as long as possible when subscribing to cable TV. We always got pushback from our two older boys, but they learned to live with this. Today, when my adult children and I reflect on those good old days, we only talk about the great memories we shared doing things as a family, and the topic of generic brand clothes or other things rarely comes up.

Move into a Problem-Solving Mode

Another benefit of maintaining a constant attitude of gratitude is that it removes you from a complaining or whining mode and keeps you consistently prepared in a solution-seeking mode. For example, when the new water park opened, our children all wanted to go, but this was over our budget. As a result, we sat down as a family and told them to offer up other ideas or activities we could do together. Since we are so lucky to live in Hawaii, the natural solution was to have a beach day, which was completely free and just as much fun. As a family, you are more likely to come up with a mutually agreed-upon solution. Everyone feels happier about this process, and it develops skills for our children to utilize in the future as adults.

Be Kind to Everyone

In this home atmosphere of gratitude, the environment should be more conducive to speaking kindly to one another and expressing gratefulness. Sometimes, the people we love the most are those we are not so lovely to because there is a comfort zone there. They are family and will love you no matter how you speak or treat them; however, when trying to cultivate those warm, fuzzy, close relationships, it never hurts to try extra hard to be cordial and courteous, just like you would behave with a stranger. The more you practice at home, the more likely you will take this attitude to your workplace or school. This attitude of gratitude can be contagious, so share it with everyone you encounter, including strangers.

Count Your Blessings

In many ways, having a positive attitude of abundance is about being mindful of the many blessings in our wonderful country. We take living in the United States for granted. I recall conversations I had with my maternal grandparents from China, who immigrated to Hawaii. They crossed the Pacific Ocean in search of a better life and had heard about the numerous great opportunities available here. They were laborers with no formal education, but within one generation, my mother attended college on the mainland and earned her master's degree in social work in the 1940s. I am so grateful to my grandparents from China, and I appreciate their courage and sacrifice in seeking a better life in a new foreign land. Even though our country is currently going through some turbulent times, I still believe it is the greatest country in the world, and I am so grateful to be a United States citizen.

One of the best ways to appreciate all your blessings is to write them down in a daily gratitude journal. Acknowledging one or two things you are grateful for daily can help prepare and strengthen you to deal with challenging situations. It's a simple way to focus on the positive aspects of your life. By writing in a gratitude journal, you are forcing yourself to tune in to the good things in your life, which you might otherwise take for granted. Scientific studies in positive psychology now demonstrate that keeping a gratitude journal helps you record your memories and find self-expression, while also benefiting your health. The conclusions of the studies indicate that journaling helps reduce stress, improve immune function, maintain a sharp memory, boost mood, and enhance emotional well-being. As a family activity, consider doing a daily gratitude journal and share your daily excerpts. You can also use your daily excerpts during "family talk about the day" and have each family member share their gratitude for that day.

Engaging the entire family in frequent discussions of gratitude will make everyone happier and help them appreciate the good things happening in everyone's lives. When you visit the abundance, you cannot help but feel contented with what you already have. At the end of our lives, we will not wish we had more things, but rather, we will be grateful for the strong relationships we have cultivated over the years with our family and friends.

CHAPTER 11

KEEP THE PASSION BURNING

Have a Winning Mindset

From a very young age, I have always been highly competitive. I always liked to win, perhaps because I was the second child yearning for my parents' attention, or because I was sandwiched between two brothers. Whether in school or outdoors on the playground, I tried my best to win and succeeded. The problem with this is that once people know what you are capable of, they expect to see the same result repeatedly. In my younger years, I felt like an average person who just tried harder than most, always hoping people wouldn't discover my secret. This proved a pretty good philosophy; my dad helped reinforce it throughout my life.

My Role Model

My dad was such an inspiration in my life. His parents, my paternal grandparents, immigrated to the United States from China and settled in Hawaii in the early 1900s. With very little English and education, they started a small store business in the Palama district of Honolulu. My dad told me stories of how my grandparents would wake up early in the morning to bake little pork buns called *manaupua* and then carry large containers of these on their shoulders around the parks and neighborhood, yelling out, "Manaupua for sale!" This hard work paid off and helped them raise my dad, his four brothers, and one older sister.

My dad was very fortunate to attend a young men's Catholic school, St. Louis High School, and he gained an excellent education at this men-only Catholic institution. Dad never officially had his graduation ceremony because World War II was in full swing. On June 14th, one day after his eighteenth birthday, he signed up for the U.S. Army. He was assigned to desk duties and never saw any action on the combat field, as the war ended soon after he enlisted. With the G.I. Bill after his service, my dad was accepted to the Massachusetts Institute of Technology, a prestigious East Coast college. Many of his classmates also attended other Ivy League colleges, like Harvard, but my dad felt happy to be at MIT. He received his master's degree in Civil engineering, with a specialization in structural engineering, a new field of expertise at that time.

I remember my dad telling stories about how he wasn't the most brilliant student, but he tried his best. He was my role model, and I admired his courage, persistence, and dedication. As a young girl, I knew everything was possible if you tried. I always believed that no matter what the outcome, I would have no regrets if I did my best.

This shaped the way I approached everything in my life. I genuinely believe that to have and maintain success, talent is only a small part of the equation. Instead, hard work, perseverance, and determination are the key to success.

Parents Are the Key to Success

At the family workshops I have conducted over the years, I am always proud of my participants, who have diligently attended sessions, completed their homework, and achieved numerous goals for themselves and their families. I then feel the most challenging part is at hand: maintaining sustained success. Whenever I see my patients and their families in the office or out and about, I always ask how things are going. This answer ultimately depends on how engaged and involved the parents are. The children are still young and do not fully grasp the lifetime benefits of their new healthy habits. So, as parents or guardians of the family, the adults must continue to take the lead.

The family talk times you have established must be continued on a weekly or, preferably, daily basis. Communication is key to reminding one another of the family's goal for the week or month and hearing about the progress other members are making along the way. Accountability, even by children, is a good motivator to keep adults on their toes.

I remember our "talk about the day" family discussions every night, during which everyone could feel free to bring up any topic of debate. I never knew what topics would be brought up. Some examples include when my children were growing up; they were the only ones in the neighborhood not receiving allowances, the unfairness of assigned chores, and the difficulty of getting permission to extend their bedtime hours, among others.

I sometimes dreaded these "talk about the day" sessions because they could last a long time, depending on the topic. I would be so tired and have a million things to do, but as I look back on these family discussions, it was one of the few times of the day when we could reconnect as a family. As the parents and leaders of the family, we would always end our discussions with "We will take this under advisement," but nothing was promised. My husband and I would later sit down and discuss the recent debate, considering whether it made sense to adjust it as needed, especially when the children grew older. The point is that when these family discussions are a regular part of the daily routine, everyone will feel that their input is valuable, and trust and respect will be gained. Allowing the older kids more privileges was always challenging with four children, but they had to earn them and prove themselves worthy.

Over the years, being a parent has been an on-the-job learning experience that neither medical school nor pediatric residency prepared me for. However, I know that regular communication and family talk time keep everyone in touch and make them much happier. Therefore, as time marches on, pause and reflect on the steady progress everyone is making on this journey toward healthier habits. If someone stands out and leads the charge with exceptional progress, recognize and reward them. It is easy to get down on oneself or others when they fail or mess up, but be mindful of positive behaviors and progress. Again, it takes time to focus on the present moment, especially when you are in one of these family talks. It is so easy to start drifting into the future, thinking about things to do, or looking back on past regrets. Still, the children will know and appreciate your undivided attention once you listen and contribute as the leader.

Building Memories for a Lifetime

It is funny how memories work. As I look back on those times as a young, overwhelmed working mom, I quickly recall the happy times we all shared as a family. These include family bike rides, family trips, staycations, Easter egg hunts, Christmases spent together, and many more family activities. I know that there were many days of fatigue, worry, trying to balance the tight budget, and tense discussions on how we should spend our money, among other things. However, the bottom line is that what mattered most was the relationships, bonding, and memories we shared as a family unit. This was the glue that helped us get through tough times. Once again, it was the perseverance, hard work, and the routines we established helped each one of us succeed. I know that it can work for you and your family, too.

Many times, my husband and I have questioned whether we are parenting correctly. The children were all different, and we always had to be flexible and adaptable while still maintaining consistency. We wanted them to grow up to be hardworking, kind, and respectful individuals who could contribute to society and make it a better place as adults. I am happy to report that, for the most part, we accomplished this task. Now that they are all in their thirties, it feels good to say, "mission accomplished". I try to share with the friends and families I work with that children are truly a gift from God, but they are only on loan to us for a short time. When they are with us, we are responsible for shaping them into well-controlled and disciplined adults. They will become their best and ultimately be happy and fulfilled individuals.

But just like everything worthwhile, it takes daily determination and patience to see the results you strive for. My parting thought is to continue working hard as a family and never give up. Your family depends on you to lead the way. When you make a mistake, remember that there's always another day to start over. I can tell you from experience that your children will thank you later for setting boundaries, spending time talking to them, and, most of all, not giving up on them or yourself.

CHAPTER 12

OOPS, WE ARE ONLY HUMAN

Obstacles Are with You at Every Season in Your Life

As a young, optimistic pre-medical student at the University of Hawai'i at Mānoa, I was suddenly thrust into a huge culture shock. As a freshman, I sat in large, theater-style rooms, sometimes filled with 100 to 200 students. Since I graduated from Maryknoll High School, a small, private Catholic high school with classes of no more than twenty-five students, this was a new experience for me. Everywhere I turned, it seemed like everyone wanted to be a doctor.

The first semester in college was brutally difficult, and several times, I confided in my dad that I wanted to quit. Through encouragement from family and friends who believed in me, I was able to adjust and survive despite the numerous obstacles. At the age of twenty, I was blessed to be accepted to the UH John A. Burns School of Medicine with an "early decision" at the start of my third year as a college senior. I felt relieved to be on my way and fulfilling my life goal. But life has a fun way of presenting you with new and even bigger obstacles.

That first year of medical school was another year of major adjustments. We were in classes from 8:00 a.m. to 5:00 p.m., and we were fed massive amounts of information daily. We also spent many hours in the anatomy lab, dissecting our cadavers and studying late into the evening. We even wore white coats in our first year of medical school and had to act like real doctors, seeing patients. These were just a few things expected of us in that first grueling year. It seemed like there was an exam every week, and I tried to keep up with everyone else. My classmates were wonderful, and we all helped one another; however, I swear I had never met so many knowledgeable people in a single class.

After this first traumatic semester, I went to the dean of students, Dr. Benjamin Young, to tell him that maybe medicine was not for me. Thankfully, he told me many students feel this way and urged me to push through. Each year that followed in medical school presented new challenges, but I kept my ultimate lifetime goal in mind and persevered. As my career progressed, increasingly larger obstacles continued to present themselves, even after I completed medical school. When you think you've gotten through the worst, you realize you haven't seen anything yet.

And so it was, at the start of my pediatric residency training at Columbus Children's Hospital, that I was now officially a physician. Still, there was so much to learn and experience. I was on call every third night, witnessed death every week, assumed many responsibilities that required split-second decisions, and much more. There is no question that I learned a lot, but even more surprises were in store for me as I opened my private practice office in Gentry Waipio, Oahu, alongside my husband and business partner.

I share this story to tell you that anything worth fighting for will not be easy. I have learned that you must invest time, effort, and hard work daily. I found that setting a goal helps you approach each day with a clear focus. In other words, don't quit; show up daily and seek help and encouragement from others. Many years ago, a politician made the saying popular that "it takes a village" to help raise a child. I now look back and see how many families and friends helped me on my journey, even when I felt like quitting. I will be forever grateful to those people who truly believed in me.

Stay Focused

Never forget that obstacles will present themselves at every opportunity; therefore, keep your goals clear in mind. Stay focused on your daily tasks and view problems as opportunities for learning and problem- solving. When you have that mindset, you become the winner. Little weekly victories will boost your confidence, knowing you are one step closer to achieving your goal of better health. Keep everyone engaged with food planning, shopping, and prepping so you won't succumb to the easier and more convenient fast food from the microwave. As parents, keep the excitement going by including fresh, new ideas. Every week, sit down, choose a new recipe, and get everyone involved in the shopping, prepping, and cooking. Start a new garden and try planting herbs or another vegetable, such as lettuce. Have a friendly competition with your family to see who can walk the most steps over the weekends. Remember, don't read every single health articles or fad diets that come up in magazines or social media but stick with the basic information you have learned in this program. Remember, moderation is a good word to have, and say it often, as it allows you to reward yourself occasionally.

Pick Each Other Up

Everyone should be reminded to conduct daily family talks and discuss the ongoing progress each person is making. If someone starts losing interest, reel them back in. This might be the perfect time for everyone to review the goal-setting chapter or sit down for a family session where you can all share your current progress. Perhaps a new goal could be set, or a previously enjoyed family activity could be reintroduced to maintain the momentum moving forward. Again, the magic of this program is that no one is alone in this journey, and if someone is struggling, pick them up and be a source of encouragement. When I conducted these family sessions in my office, I tried to remind everyone at each session that they should expect days when they don't feel like doing anything healthy. Remember, it's not about feeling like doing it; it's about the actions we take.

The Five-Second Rule

I recently came across a novel way of overcoming the hurdle of doing something, even when you don't "feel" like it. I have tried it myself many times, which has helped me accomplish goals I never thought possible. This concept, known as the "Five Second Rule," was introduced by Mel Robbins and has proven highly successful for many people. No, this is not the rule, which states that if a piece of food falls on the floor and is picked up within five seconds, you may still eat it. Instead, this rule keeps us from hesitating and catapults us into action. Our brains are wired to avoid doing things that seem scary, complex, or frightening, so when you hesitate, your brain wakes up to magnify the problem. This phenomenon is known as the spotlight effect, which occurs in under five seconds. Therefore, by counting backward–five, four, three, two, one–your brain has no time to stop you, and you immediately catapult into action.

Using this five-second rule, you can go from idea to action. You know clearly what you want, the goal is in mind, and the only thing left to do is to push forward with courage and positivity. By using this five-second rule, you force yourself to be in the present moment, not regretting the past and not worrying about the future. It empowers you to feel excited about taking the right action and putting aside the real enemy, fear. The "Five Second Rule" by Mel Robbins is one of the top ten TED Talks ever viewed, and this method of moving into action is used worldwide. In one of my workshops, a family member of mine used this technique to lead a daily family walk. There was never a day when every single family member felt like walking, but they all shouted "5, 4, 3, 2, 1" in unison, and everyone put on their shoes and set out to walk. When this walk was completed, they all felt so proud of themselves for accomplishing what seemed like an almost impossible task.

Remember, you are in control of the thoughts and actions in your life. You must decide on the most critical tasks to accomplish today and prioritize them. Using the five-second rule helps you to stay hyper-aware and focused on your present goal. If you want to make changes now, you must beat the fear that is real and in front of you. Instead of thinking about fear, think of excitement and challenge. Adults are responsible for "parenting themselves" because no one will tell us what to do. Once we understand this and accept the challenge, we can move forward toward making our dreams come true.

The Secret of a Lifetime of Success

This journey you are taking toward better health is not an easy one and will require hard work. In a recent study, Angela Lee Duckworth discusses her search to find the key components of success. She wanted to see the secret to success. She looked at West Point graduates, Ivy League school graduates, spelling bee winners, prosperous businesspeople, and many others from various fields. She concluded that grit and self-control were the two most critical predictive variables in their real-world performances. Thomas Edison says that "genius is mostly just perspiration." The conclusion is that our most important talent in life is working hard, not giving up, and practicing even when it does not feel like fun. Another way of looking at this is that you need to develop mental toughness to achieve any goals in your life. Thus, mental toughness is built daily through your small wins, like a muscle being challenged and growing every day. We must remember to focus on small habits, be consistent, stick to the schedule, and forget about the results. When you slip up, pick yourself up and get back on track. If you can maintain consistency in this mindset, you can accomplish anything.

Seeking the Help You Need

One final note to close this chapter on obstacles and roadblocks. As someone who has personally been through two major depressive episodes in my life, I never thought in a million years that this would happen to me. This is a real illness; just like any other illness, there is no shame in getting the help you need. This is my plea for you: if you are feeling extreme sadness and loss of interest in life, please do not take this lightly. This could be more than just the "blues." It could be depression, especially if it is causing you problems in your day-to-day activities. Depression is not a weakness, and you cannot simply snap out of it. Please pick up your phone now to schedule an appointment with your doctor or a mental health professional.

If you think you might hurt yourself or attempt suicide, call 9-1-1 or your local emergency number. The National Suicide Prevention Lifeline number in the United States is 1-800-273-8255 (1-800-273-TALK).

Remember, your life matters; there is help and hope for you. Reach out and call a loved one, friend, or the National Suicide Prevention Lifeline for help.

CHAPTER 13

EXCEPTIONAL FAMILY HEALTH FOR LIFE

Working Parents Can Succeed

After conducting numerous group sessions and speaking individually with my patients and their families in my office over the years, I have found that the most rewarding aspect for me is witnessing not only physical health improvements for everyone in the family but also the family unit becoming stronger and thriving once again. As a practicing pediatrician for over thirty-five years, I have witnessed firsthand the gradual erosion of the most fundamental unit in our society: the family unit. Working parents are trying their very best to keep it all together. However, our environment and technology have greatly influenced our lifestyles. I hope you come back together as a family with this program and feel connected when you work as a team. Together, everyone will be able to achieve not only health goals but also better emotional well-being.

During many sessions with parents, I have observed improved communication and increased appreciation for one another. Not only does this make all family members happy, but the children now see their parents working together as united leaders of their families. There is no longer any confusion about expectations or schedules, as everything is clear, and daily schedules are now in order. Mealtimes and bedtimes become enjoyable opportunities for family conversation, and everyone looks forward to coming home in the evening to spend quality time together.

The family leaders, parents, or guardians now feel excited about their responsibilities and the results they are seeing with these small changes. When the children see your excitement, they become excited as well. I like to call this excitement or enthusiasm "passion."

John Maxwell, who has written many books on leadership, once said, "A great leader's courage to fulfill his vision comes from passion, not position." I want each one of you, parent leaders, to get up each day thinking of new and different ways to achieve the goals of getting yourself and your family healthier. Your family is unique, so set goals that make sense for you and your family. When you move into action, show your family your energy, positivity, and passion.

It will be very contagious and soon everyone will want to follow you.

Dream Big One Step at a Time

Attempting a program like this is extremely intimidating, and the results may be uncertain. Instead, I encourage you to dream big, begin now, and be bold. Courage is doing what you are afraid of doing. Knowing that each new day is a new beginning, you can take that first step boldly and confidently. I know what it feels like – I have been there, paralyzed in that fear of mode. With the help of many, I am truly living the life I was meant to live.

A well-known Chinese saying is, "A journey of a thousand miles begins with the first step." This is so true for any journey we take. By taking small steps for continual improvement every day, they will eventually add up and become bigger things. However, you must be patient and give it time. The secret is to take small, itty, bitty steps that will eventually lead to those giant leaps. When you take small baby steps, you cannot fail, and your mind will want to keep trying a new goal. By setting small goals, your brain will bypass fear and become engaged, as it seeks success again. So, let's all become optimistic in our belief that we all have the potential for continual improvement if we do it slowly and consistently.

Opportunities to Learn and Grow

As you connect more as a family, you will learn to welcome and embrace challenges as new opportunities for everyone to learn something new. When things aren't going the way you want them to, don't be helpless, act. Acting turns worry into positive, focused energy. Be flexible and expect results to go your way. Your success in life will depend on how you deal with your failures. Continue to be passionate about your goals and strive to reach higher levels each time.

Pay It Forward

Finally, I encourage all the families I work with to share their newfound knowledge, success, and secrets for improved health with others they meet. In other words, could you pay it forward? Now that you have gained insight into better health as a family, share it freely. We influence one another, and you will become a powerful motivator for others you encounter. You are now the one who encourages others by striving to do better each day. The more you help others, the more I believe you will continue to support yourself and your family. This becomes a win-win for everyone, and it all starts with you.

The New Family Revolution

We are in a new revolution aimed at restoring the family unit. By strengthening this unit once again, you will experience improved health and enhanced emotional and spiritual well-being. The problem is that few of us are aware of this, and many families still lack an understanding of it. My hope and dream are that you and your family stay together and keep spreading the word until we turn this unhealthy trend around. Let us cherish our families and show everyone what a powerful and positive source they can be, especially when we are shaping our children. The family revolution has started with you, and I hope we can soon burst out and change the world for the better, one family at a time. Won't you join me in this happy, healthy revolution?

ACKNOWLEDGMENTS

I want to acknowledge several important individuals and groups who have supported me throughout my journey to complete this book.

First, I would like to thank my dear husband, Martin M. Arinaga, for his love and support throughout all my new adventures over the past 12 years. You are a constant source of encouragement and always see the potential in me, even when I don't. Most of all, you have deepened my relationship with God, and I am so blessed to have you at my side in life.

Thank you to my pastor, Jerry Higashi, for being my spiritual support. I appreciate your prayers and words of encouragement, especially during my despair. Your unexpected hospital visits and many talks have helped me immensely.

Thank you to my dear monthly grief support group, especially Pastor J. P., Sandy, Charlie, and Donna, for being there and helping me through my grief journey these past 15 years.

To my hardworking office staff, Danielle, Kristen, and Lori, thank you for all the late nights and the extra time you have given to help me. I could not have done it without your daily encouragement and deep belief in my movement.

To Aloha Care Health Insurance and the Aloha Care Community Intervention Program, thank you for honoring me as one of your 2019 grantees. None of this would have been possible without your support of the Hawaii Healthy Family Revolution Sessions. Thank you for investing in me and believing in me—a special thank you to Sara and Stella for helping me throughout this process. Together, we will continue to accomplish much and significantly improve the health of Hawaii, one family at a time.

To Dr. Derrin Fukuda, psychologist, and Justin Shigematsu, certified personal trainer, thank you for your valuable input and enthusiastic participation in all the sessions.

Thank you to UHA Health Insurance, its fantastic marketing department, and a massive thank you to the CEO, Howard Lee, for having the foresight to see the possibilities of new, innovative programs. I appreciate the generous support of my nonprofit organization, Walk with a Doc – Oahu, as well as Hike with a Doc, Craft with a Doc, Dance with a Doc, and Cook with a Doc, over the past 10 years.

Together, we will continue to have a profound, positive impact on many lives.

To the Queens Akoakoa Physician Organization, thank you for the privilege and honor of serving as your Pediatric Program director and for your support of my community outreach projects. You have been instrumental in helping me reach our physicians and communities. Special thanks to Whitney, Ashley, Emily, Valerie, and Lara, as well as to Susan Murray, CEO of Queens Medical Center West, for all your support.

To Walk with a Doc National Headquarters in Columbus, Ohio, especially to CEO Dr. David Sabgir and his hardworking staff, Rachel, Bryan, and Gina, as well as my dear mentor, friend, and avid Walk with a Doc supporter Dr. Annemarie Sommer, thank you for showing me what a few committed individuals can do to change the world. I love being part of your Walk with a Doc team and the movement to improve the world's health.

Thank you to my grandparents, parents, and siblings, who have loved me unconditionally and have made countless sacrifices for me. I appreciate and am grateful for everything.

To my four beautiful children – David and his wife, Cheree; Chris and his wife, Samantha; Bradley; and Stephanie Malia – thank you for your love and support, especially after the sudden and unexpected death of Dad. I am genuinely grateful for being blessed with the four of you, even though you drove me crazy at times. I know that Dad would have been so proud of the caring adults you have become. I know I am. Special thanks to my eldest son, David, for immediately stepping up and helping me establish and thrive in my private practice over the past 13 years.

Finally, I thank my awesome God for his bountiful blessings. Even in my darkest days, you have been there with me, and I will continue to give you thanks and praise. Your love endures forever, and your faithfulness continues through all generations. Let me continue to be your instrument of hope and love for others.

ABOUT THE AUTHOR

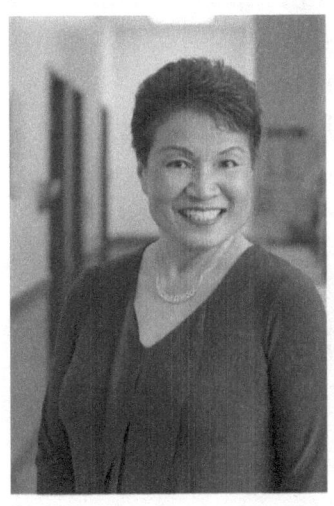

Dr. Theresa Y. Wee has been a pediatric health and wellness expert in private practice at the Wee Wellness Center for over 40 years. She completed her medical degree at the University of Hawaii John A. Burns School of Medicine and her pediatric internship, residency, and Ambulatory Fellowship at Columbus Children's Hospital (now Nationwide Children's Hospital) in Columbus, Ohio.

Dr. Wee was born and raised in Hawaii and is strongly committed to improving the health of the people there. Her non-profit organization, Walk with a Doc – Oahu, recently celebrated its ninth anniversary.

She meets weekly at Central Oahu Regional Park to educate, exercise, and encourage people to take their first step toward better health. She has also been conducting Family Obesity Sessions over the years to help families prevent, treat, and address childhood obesity.

She has also provided monthly television health tips on KHON's "Living 808 Program" for many years, as well as numerous radio segments and in-person community presentations.

In her spare time, she enjoys traveling, water aerobics, cooking, and spending time with her four children and five grandchildren. She lives in Oahu, Hawaii, with her husband, Martin M. Arinaga.

THANK YOU

Thank you so much for completing my book, *The Happy, Healthy Revolution*. I am so proud of you and hope your journey towards better health and thriving as a family continues for a lifetime.

To keep the passion alive for your entire family, continue revisiting areas in this book that seem especially challenging. This journey you are all embarking on will not happen overnight, so be patient, encourage one another, and above all, don't give up!

My hope and dream are that your entire family will enjoy improved health and better emotional and spiritual well-being. This modern revolution of returning to the family unit has begun with you; now, get out and share it with others! Together, we can change the world, one family at a time.

www.ingramcontent.com/pod-product-compliance
Lightning Source LLC
Chambersburg PA
CBHW031423120626
46545CB00006B/2241